Diagnostic Testing of Deaf Children:
The Syndrome of Dyspraxia

Diagnostic Testing of Deaf Children: The Syndrome of Dyspraxia

Dr. A. van Uden

1983

SWETS & ZEITLINGER, LISSE

CIP-GEGEVENS

Uden, A. van

Diagnostic testing of deaf children : the syndrome of
dyspraxia / A. van Uden. - Lisse : Swets & Zeitlinger. -
Ill., tab., fig.
Met lit. opg., index.
ISBN 90-265-0436-5
SISO 606.1 UDC 616.21≥616.83
Trefw. : doofheid ; spraakstoornissen.

Cover H. Veltman
Printed in the Netherlands by Offsetdrukkerij Kanters B.V., Alblasserdam
Copyright 1983 Dr. A. van Uden and Swets & Zeitlinger B.V.

ISBN 90 265 0436 5

Contents

VIII

Introductory chapter

Dysphasia in deaf children

This study is concerned with prelingually profoundly deaf children. It does not include those children who have losses of less than 95 dB (Fletcher index ISO) or those children who suffer from a so-called "ski-slope hearing loss", "low pass hearing".

1. PRELINGUAL PROFOUND DEAFNESS

By "prelingual profound deafness" is meant here, cybernetically speaking, such a hearing loss that the person is unable to hear his own voice or speech, i.e. has a greater loss than this "deafness level":

125	250	500	1000	2000	4000Hz
60	60	95	95	95	95 dB (ISO)

By "prelingual" we mean in this study: congenital. This term also applies to cases where the onset of deafness occurs during the first months of life, particularly where deafness occurs before 18 months.

It is further presupposed that the children in this study have a performance IQ of 80 or higher, and a normal memory.

2. SPECIFIC LEARNING DIFFICULTIES, ADDITIONAL TO DEAFNESS

Many deaf children in addition to being prelingually profoundly deaf also suffer from specific learning difficulties which impede satisfactory

1

development in speech and lipreading. Routine psychological testing does not indicate these difficulties. In the educational situation it is found that these children do not lipread or speak well, despite ideal educational opportunities. The question must be asked why some profoundly deaf children of average intelligence or above, fail to make adequate progress in speech and lipreading. It can also be asked why some postlingually deaf persons have difficulty in learning to lipread and may even loose their speech while others develop fluent speech, adequate lipreading, and full use of their sound perception. The answers to these questions are of the greatest importance, not only for diagnostic purposes but also in order to help the individual to benefit from educational treatment based on his specific needs.

In addition to deafness, two handicaps which endanger an oral development in deaf children have been detected. The first is a motor handicap called apraxia or dyspraxia. A factor analysis revealed that finger development (eupraxia), development of rhythm (eurhythmia), fluent speech, lipreading, and speech-hearing are a single factor. Apraxia or dyspraxia of the fingers and arhythmia or dysrhythmia involve apraxia or dyspraxia of speech including difficulty in speech-reading and speech-hearing development. However, a strength noted in children suffering from these conditions is a strong memory for simultaneously presented visual data, including the graphic form of words. This ability can be used as a support for speech and verbal development. – The second is a cognitive-motor handicap called intermodal integration disability. The ability to read normally (culexia) is based on the integration of the written and spoken form of words. This appears to be related to the quick use of word meanings (eusymbolia). A disability in this intermodal integration endangers the meaningful oral functioning and the development of reading and writing. These multiple handicaps can be detected at 3 or 4 years of age. Special tests for the detection of these handicaps have been developed.

The syndrome of dyspraxia/apraxia in deaf children and adults is the main topic of this book. The syndrome of the intermodal disability will be the main topic of a second study.

3. THE DEAF A HOMOGENEOUS GROUP?

It is clear that the deaf cannot be viewed as a homogeneous group. In the hearing population there is variability in such traits as level of intellectual functioning, socio-economic-cultural status and background, sensori-motor, and emotional functioning. This variability is also found in the deaf and often in a greater degree than in the hearing population. It must also be said that some deaf children live in circumstances and in environments where opportunities for adequate educational treatment is poor, and where they do not get those opportunities which are necessary for their full human development. The reason for the many educational failures is that the lack of such opportunities is not recognised in time, because the specific capacities, both positive and negative, of the children are not adequately diagnosed.

It is generally accepted that all deaf children need to learn to talk via speech-reading and speech-hearing, according to the best of their ability, oral language being their first or their second language. We know that such an oral development in many deaf children is not satisfactory, even after many years of schooling. The reason is not only a lack of the external circumstances needed (acceptance process on the part of the parents, parent and school cooperation, qualification of teachers, etc.) but also additional disabilities in the child. Several of these disabilities are clear enough and it is possible to take corrective measures in time.

These disabilities might be considered in terms of:
a. Emotional functioning: hysteric and hysteroid tendencies, pathological weaknesses in concentration, autism, hyperactivity.
b. Motor functioning: spasm, athetosis, choreo-athetosis, choreiformity, ataxia, and severe clumsiness.
c. Cognitive functioning: mental deficiency, difficulty with memory, perceptual disturbance.

The importance of the exact diagnosis of the memory function must be emphasised as it is an area often neglected by psychologists, neurologists, and psychiatrists. Yet, a disability of memory seems to be the most dangerous and significant of all. A precise diagnosis of the variability of memory functioning with its typical profile, differing from child to child, is fundamental for a well-planned educational programme.

There are other additional disabilities, however, which are less striking to the untrained eye and can only be detected by a careful diagnosis. Dyspraxia, the subject of the present study, is one of these.

In order to give some indication of the direction and orientation of this study it may be helpful to consider some basic concepts and the relationship between dyspraxia/apraxia and other disorders in deaf children.

4. CHILDREN WHO HAVE DIFFICULTY ACQUIRING
   SPEECH, AND DYSSYMBOLIC CHILDREN

Those of us acquainted with deaf children know that there are a lot of deaf children who have difficulty acquiring speech and that there are also quite a number of dyssymbolic ones among the deaf population, both children and adults. We may ask the questions: Is this a disturbance, a

3

disability? And if so, which one? How can it be detected and at what age?

It often happens that a child of average intelligence or above who has been receiving excellent oral education and systematic training in speech fails to acquire adequate speech even after three or four years training. This represents a great disappointment for the parents, and indeed the child himself. One of the aims of this study is to show how such disappointing developments can be prevented.

We may now consider some preliminary concepts related to this study.

5. DYSPHASIA IN DEAF CHILDREN

Two meanings of dys- and aphasia have been noted in the literature dealing with this topic. The first is indicated by a kind of apraxia, clumsiness, and has been recognised for a long time in patients suffering from motor aphasia, described as a disturbance in the "body relation-gnosis" (Prick and Calon, 1950), or the control of the body scheme. The terms "dyspraxia" and "apraxia *of speech*" have been used in this respect. Eupraxia can be defined operationally as:

The quick finding of the members (*articulators*) needed for an action or a speech act.

The terminology of dysphasia and aphasia is also used in another context, namely that of the so-called "Gerstmann Syndrome" (1927) including echolalic, dyslectic and dysgraphic traits which can be summarised as a disturbance in sensori-motor integration. These two kinds of dysphasia and aphasia, namely, the apraxia of speech and the speech and language integration disturbance, should not be too detached from each other, although they are different. Perhaps we may speak of a shifting of emphasis, on the one hand the emphasis on the motor pro-gramming (Lashley, 1951) and on the other hand the emphasis on the intermodal integration (in the perception, imagination, and memory). An example may further illustrate this point:

We may take an example from the training of deaf children: the so-called "planting" of a word such as "flower" in the deaf child. In this example the following aspects are important:
1. the full experience of a flower (its feel, smell, to pick it, to use it for different purposes),
2. lipreading,
3. speech hearing, including vibration-feeling of speech,
4. speech programming in the brain and the muscles,
5. reading and writing the word,
6. widening the experience and interpreting pictures etc.

These aspects are illustrated in Fig. 1.

4

Figure 1. An integrated sensori-motor Gestalt.

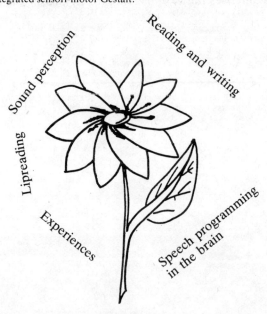

A disturbance of any one of these aspects hampers the "Gestalt formation" and therefore the eusymbolia of the word flower; e.g. when the
speech programming is clumsy and/or the written form of the word has
not been imprinted clearly enough, the child may forget the word, mix it
up with other words, etc.

It can happen, however, that the integration as such is disturbed, e.g.
the speech programming is correct, the memory for the written form of
the word is also correct, yet both forms do not integrate. In this case the
Gestalt formation does not develop as smoothly as it should. We may
describe this integration disability as an "integrative dyslexia", in which
the graphic form of the word does not evoke its spoken form. This may
lead to a kind of "integrative dysgraphia", a condition in which the child
cannot write down a word spoken by himself even after considerable
training. The effect of such an intermodal integration disturbance goes
even deeper: the experiences of the flower do not integrate strongly
enough with the language code, i.e. the words are not integrated or
associated with their meaning quickly enough. This causes difficulties in
the finding of the correct words and in the correct interpretation of the
word (dyssymbolia) and, in some very pronounced cases, asymbolia for
verbal language.

5

Figure 2 summarises the two meanings of dysphasia and aphasia:

Figure 2.

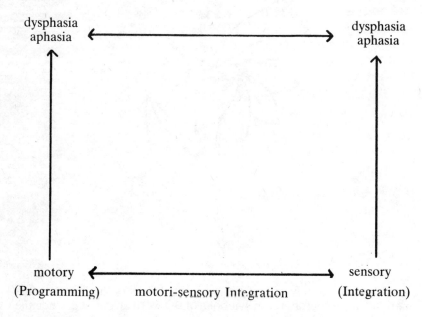

6. SOME PHENOMENA IN HEARING ADULTS

Fucci et al. (1977) investigated the reaction of normal, hearing and speaking young adults, when the auditory control of their speech had been taken away by using a masking noise. They found that some subjects did not show a speech disturbance at all, but other subjects definitely did. They rightly concluded that the *speech programming* of these latter ones must be typically dependent upon auditory control, which was not the case in the former. There must be assumed a kind of motor speech programming (in my opinion in the same sense as Lashley, 1951), which does not have the same strength in all normally hearing speakers. Sands et al. (1978) have shown that in some patients suffering from aphasia due to brain damage a dyspraxia and/or apraxia of speech was a part of the syndrome.

Luria (1966) speaks of a "simultaneous" and "successive *integrative* process" of speech, which integration can be disturbed by brain damage. This disturbance can appear at the perceptual level, the "mnestic" level

6

and/or the intellectual level. Brookshire (1978) has shown that an intermodal, sensori-motor integration disturbance in patients suffering from aphasia can be tested by means of the "Token-test" (DeRenzi and Vignolo, 1962). Cf. also Broesterhuizen et al. (1980).

7. CONGENITAL DYSPHASIA AND APHASIA IN NORMALLY HEARING CHILDREN

Breuer and Weuffen (1975, 1977) have shown an interdependency or interaction between disturbances of rhythmic development, of memory for speech and dysgrammaticism, in normally hearing children of 3-8 years of age. See also Elstner and Karlstad (1978) and Lotzman (1979). Some paedagogues of Amsterdam have humorously and meaningfully called these *dyspraxic*, sometimes even apraxic, very clumsy children: "the small demolishers"! Actually in a normally hearing child the dyspraxia must be very very strong, much stronger than in a deaf child, before an aphasia or dysphasia may appear. It may appear sooner, when the auditory memory is not strong enough, resulting into a disturbed memory for speech and dysgrammaticism. This dysgrammaticism (e.g. "Bump me! My arm! Peter bump!") obviously originates from the fact that the child, after two or three words, has forgotten how he started his utterance, and therefore is unable to structure it in a longer grammatical sentence. These normally hearing children do behave very clumsily indeed.

Das et al. (1975, 1978), following the theory of Luria (1966), have shown a sensori-motor *integration* disturbance in very many dyslexic normally hearing children. Senf (1972) even thinks that all learning disabilities are only a sensori-motor integration disturbances: "Disorders in information processing and information integrating systems". Other researchers say the same, although in other terms, e.g. Ross (1976) "disability to recode and reorganize information", Vellutino (1977) and Torgesen (1979, quoted by Wong 1979), "encoding disorders", "verbal deficit". The last writer describes these children as "more impulsive", "easily distracted", etc.

8. HISTORICAL NOTES FROM THE INSTITUTE FOR THE DEAF SINT MICHIELSGESTEL

a. The detection of the phenomena
The publication of reliable intelligence scales (e.g. Ewing with the Wechsler Test, 1957; Snijders-Oomen Non-verbal Intelligence Scale, 1958) brought attention to the *problem*:

7

How is it possible that some deaf children, with normal, sometimes even high intelligence, who apparently behave very skilfully in gymnastics and sports, do not acquire speech unless with great difficulty and clumsily, sometimes not at all, and do not learn to lipread and to use their auditory remnants satisfactorily?

We started to investigate this phenomenon more deeply and carefully in 1967, in deaf children with normal intelligence and who had been instructed by expert teachers and speech teachers. We followed the course of the eupraxia. We studied the difference between so-called transitive and *intransitive movements* (see below). "Transitive movements" are those movements which use some material towards an objective, e.g. dressing oneself, moulding and kneading plasticine, drawing, building, constructing, most of the movements in gymnastics and sports, etc. The subject controls these movements mainly because the material evokes them: the nature of the material helps the subject to control these transitive movements. A child, even being clumsy, may execute those movements skilfully, especially if he is intelligent and able to compensate for his clumsiness; he may even appear to be very skilful, e.g. in sports. "Intransitive movements" do not use material: e.g. dancing, and last but not least speaking. It became clear to us that it was almost impossible to detect our "clumsy speakers" by means of tests for transitive movements, e.g. for dressing apraxia, but they became easier to detect by using tests for intransitive movements, such as tests for eurhythmia, for movements of the fingers, for speech. See e.g. Bergès and Lézine (1963), Zazzo (1964). The Oseretsky-Test, revised by Bruininks (1978), has several subtests now for intransitive movements.

By means of these tests the control of the body scheme, the "body relation-gnosis" (Prick and Calon, 1950) can easily be detected. Dyspraxia *is* actually a disturbance of this control of the body scheme. At the time of our investigation, 15 years ago, we had to develop our own tests.

A multiple correlation between, on the one side, speech-, lipreading- and speech-hearing-development and on the other, scores of our eupraxia tests, including eurhythmia tests, appeared again and again in different groups.

Another phenomenon appeared, namely in cognitive behavior:

On the average the dyspraxic and motorily dysphasic deaf children showed a better memory for colours, pictures, bead-patterns, i.e. for simultaneously presented visual data. But when they had to imitate and to memorize successively presented visual data, such as pictures in succession, paper-folding patterns, block-tapping patterns etc., they scored too low on the average in comparison with the eupraxic deaf children. We published this in 1970 and 1972, see chapter V. In 1974 a polar factor could be shown, see chapter VI. We have called this inter-

8

dependency of motor and cognitive aspects of behaviour: "The *syndrome of dyspraxia* in deaf children", and will describe it in the next sections of this book.

The *integration* of the written form of words and their spoken form is a very important aspect in the didactics of deaf children. We therefore developed a "reading integration test", standardized for deaf children of 7-13 years of age (1968). Twenty-five words are used, one-syllabic through five-syllabic ones. The child is tested individually. Each word has been type-written on a card, and this card is shown to the child for 3 seconds. The child then has to pronounce the word from memory. The correct syllabes are counted. Immediately after the series of 25 words have been presented in this way, the same series is presented to the child again, but now the child has not to pronounce the word, but to write it down from memory. The standardization and the application of this test revealed another learning difficulty in deaf children, termed by us "sensori-motor integration disturbance". Typically enough the second part of the test (visual-visual, no clear integration problem) is executed by some children much better than the first part (visual-articulatory, a clear integration problem). Children showing a disability in this respect showed the same disability in reading notes of music when playing our "blow-organs", and in executing rhythmic movements according to graphic rhythmic symbols, e.g. ●●, ●●●, ● ● etc. See p. 103. (This part of our investigation is as yet incomplete.)

We found the following:

- There are some dyspraxic deaf children suffering from a sensori-motor integration disturbance in addition to deafness and dyspraxia;
- there are deaf children suffering only from dyspraxia, without an integration problem;
- there are deaf children suffering only from a sensori-motor integration disturbance, not from dyspraxia;
- there are deaf children not suffering from either of these two dangerous disturbances.

We started an exact observation of the daily behaviour of the children with a sensori-motor integration disturbance. In 1978 we were able to compose an inventory by means of which house-parents and teachers are able to describe carefully the behaviour of the children. The inventory comprises three parts (see van Uden, 1979):

- non-verbal behaviour, from early years through to adulthood;
- non-verbal and verbal behaviour from 5-years of age through to adulthood;
- higher verbal behaviour, from 8 years of age through to adulthood.

A relationship between "integrative eulexia-dyslexia-alexia" and "eusymbolia-dyssymbolia-asymbolia" appeared. For that reason we have termed these children: our "dyssymbolic deaf".

9

Now we are at the stage that we can warn of these two disturbances, either singly or both together, at the ages of 3-4 years.

b. A "diagnostic centre"

Since about 1970 our home training-service, the "changing-class" for deaf children of 2-3 years of age, and our preschool for deaf children of 4-6 years of age, co-operate as one longitudinal diagnostic centre. By means of this our Institute is able to diagnose reliably, to what extent and by what methods the deaf child concerned can be educated orally and verbally.

For this specialized and sophisticated diagnosis of learning disabilities in deaf children the following persons co-operate:

A team of teachers of the deaf, the respective heads of home training and preschool, two orthopaedagogues, two psychologists and one psychological associate. All children are investigated throughout, and the investigations are repeated in a longitudinal way at least three times before a decision for one of the special departments of the Institute is taken. Factors concerning the decision are not only the motor-cognitive behaviour "in abstracto" of the child, but his total functioning, including his character and memory functions; even the co-operation of the parents and the ability of the teachers and educators available may play a part.

This Institute has three departments for its deaf children of normal intelligence:

- the main departments, i.e. for deaf children without heavy multiple disturbances;
- a department for moderately dysphasic deaf children;
- a department for heavily dysphasic, sometimes even aphasic deaf children, who need fingerspelling in addition to speech, lipreading and speech-hearing (as much as they can), as a support for the mainly graphic conversation, for development of speech, and for communication among themselves.

In the years 1974 through 1979 95 prelingually profoundly deaf children with normal performal intelligence of the ages $2^1/_2$-6 years passed through our diagnostic centre, mentioned above, see Table 1.

c. The syndrome of dyspraxia and its treatment

The syndrome of dyspraxia of deaf children indicates that the child clearly suffers from dyspraxia or apraxia with dysrhythmia or arhythmia, and that the child, his memory as such being normal, shows a typical profile of a strong memory for simultaneously presented visual data, and a relatively weak one for successively presented visual data.

Most important, as always, is conversation, even in the home training. We mention especially the importance, better to say the necessity, of

Table 1.
Diagnosis of 95 prelingually profoundly deaf children with normal performance intelligence 2¹/₂-6 years of age, 1974-1979.
The decision for a special department has been taken at the average age of 5¹/₂ years.

Diagnosis	Main department	Department for moderately dysphasic deaf children	Department for heavily dysphasic and aphasic deaf children (finger-spelling with speech)	Total
No heavy learning disability	55%	–	–	55%
Only dyspraxia	7%	5%	3%	15%
Only sensori-motory integration disturbance	6%	1%	1%	8%
Both dyspraxia and integration disturbance	3%	12%	7%	22%
Total	71%	18%	11%	100%

"depositing" the spoken language used into the deaf children's diaries, with the use of speechballoons (van Uden, 1978). The more a child suffers from dyspraxia, the more these deposits become important for him. We may even have to develop "graphic conversation" for some of the most heavy cases.

Special measures will be necessary for the development of speech (van Uden, 1974, 1980): a "reactive method", Kern's method ("Tast-Fühl-Struktur" "tactually felt structure" 1958), and sometimes the strongly analytical method of Vatter (see e.g. McGinnis, 1963).
    As soon as the child becomes mature enough (may be 4¹/₂ years of age), a strong integration of the written and the spoken form of the words must be developed. All of this can be done very playfully. From 5 years of age it is certainly possible to start work using the typewriter, with the Communicator (Canon). Even preschool children like to play with it and it is a help in the imprinting of the written form of the words, and for the copying of them. This strong memory of the written form of the words becomes a strong support for speech. Many of these children are

not able to co-ordinate their speech, and certainly not when it becomes more complex, without this graphic support.

This graphic conversation and learning to typewrite may grow in such a way that in later years a "group-graphic-aid" can be used.

An important help in developing lipreading is a training in lipreading from themselves. This can be accomplished by making the child speak words and sentences into the camera of a video-recorder, and get the child to lipread from his own speech on the monitor afterwards. We found significant gains in lipreading (1970, 1974). The same with auditory training (van Uden, 1955).

A kind of "kinetic therapy" is necessary too, with playful training in eurhythmia, music, dance, expressive movements and planning behaviour.

d. A few extremely difficult cases of apraxia of speech

The few deaf children who are so aphasic that they need fingerspelling are termed by us "deaf dactyl children". The graphic conversation method is used for all these children (cf. Al. Graham Bell, 1884).

We may show now the results of just one class, a class of four children (1980), 17-19 years of age. They have been mainly educated graphically for more than 10 years. They converse among themselves using speech and finger spelling (the one-hand alphabet). Ten years ago these children were as yet unable to speak at all or only very clumsily and backwardly.

The following information can be given (names are pseudonyms):
James came to our school rather late, at the age of 8 years, and had not had any special training before. He suffers heavily from the syndrome of apraxia, described above. We had to start immediately with finger spelling, speech and graphic conversation.

Mary suffers from a full acoustic agnosia, together with the apraxia syndrome. She had been educated and trained in a pedological institute, without result. She too came to our school at the age of 8 years, and has been treated in the same way as James.

Annmary has been educated by our home-training service and in our preschool. She is slightly choreo-athetoid and suffers both from the syndrome of apraxia and sensori-motor integration disturbance. Shortly after preschool she was taken in by our special department for strongly aphasic deaf children.

Corry too was treated by our home-training and in the preschool. She suffers from the syndrome of apraxia together with sensori-motor integration disturbance, the latter being heavier than the first. She was treated in the same way as Annmary.

At this time, after a long treatment, a mainly oral conversation is possible, but very often supported by typewriting, and sometimes by finger spelling too.

After two years of training, when the children were about 10-12 years of age, it became possible to measure their verbal intelligence *graphically*, for the first time. Their performance intelligence had been measured before, and they scored an average of 117 (100 to 130). The verbal questions, directions and tasks, to be given orally to normally hearing children and adults, were presented to these children graphically:

For example: "What is the capital of the Netherlands?" – "In what way are a *rose* and a *daisy* alike? How are they the same?" – "Count these apples!" – "What does *bread* mean?" etc. The child (tested individually) had to read the questions or directions, and to write down his answers.

The Wechsler Intelligence Scale was taken (Belgian and Dutch standardization). This measurement was repeated every two years (by our psychological associate, L. Merken). The results are shown in Table 2:

Table 2

Names (pseudonyms)	Multiple handicap	Audiogram (Fletcher-index)	Has had home training	Has had preschool	Age	Used Wechsler Intelligence Test WISC 10-15 years and WAIS 15;11 years and older:	
						Performal IQ	Verbal IQ
James	syndrome of apraxia	105 dB	no	no	1. 10;0	96	50
					2. 12;3	104	98
					3. 13;5	101	101
					4. 15;0	102	108
					5. 17;8	110	108
Corry	syndrome of apraxia and sensori-motor integration disturbance	115 dB	yes	yes	1. 10;10	128	50
					2. 13;3	131	66
					3. 14;5	130	72
					4. 15;11	120	75
					5. 18;7	126	96
Mary	syndrome of apraxia and acoustic agnosia	? agnosia	no	no	1. ...	...	...
					2. 15;9	120	75
					3. 16;10	128	96
					4. 18;4	128	96
					5. 21;0	124	100
Annmary	syndrome of apraxia, choreo-athetosis and sensori-motor integration disturbance	109 dB	r.o	yes	1. 11;11	120	68
					2. 14;4	123	76
					3. 15;6	121	86
					4. 17;0	126	89
					5. 19;8	130	102

14

We can summarize the results in a diagram, see Figure 3.

Figure 3.

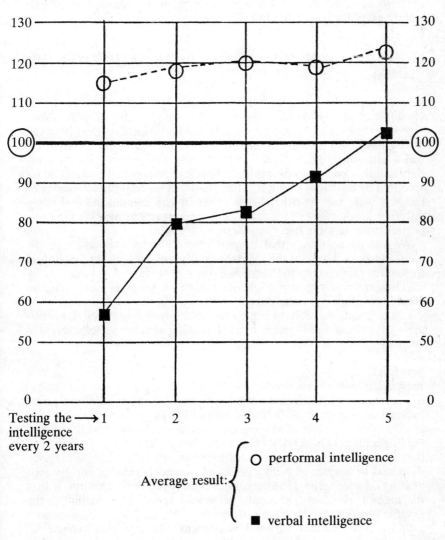

Testing the ⟶ intelligence every 2 years

Average result:
O performal intelligence

■ verbal intelligence

It may be clear from these data that the performal intelligence is fairly constant through the 8-year span, but that the *verbal* intelligence increases with age.

These children have been learning English in addition to Dutch mainly graphically, for the last 3 years.

9. THE VALUE OF THE GRAPHIC INFORMATION FOR THE DEAF

Several researches (Gates, 1971; White, 1972; Caccamise, 1976: Stuckless et al., 1976) have shown clearly enough that *graphic information* is the best and the most reliable one for all kinds of deaf persons, if they have only learned to understand the written word: for children and adults, for prelingually and postlingually deaf persons, for the multiply handicapped and non-multiply handicapped ones. This fact can be accepted by devotees of different methods, by us who are advocates of the oral way, and by others who swear by the manual method using different kinds of sign language. Such an agreement may be very important coming after two centuries of discussion.

We should be aware that graphic information is increasing in the western world. Think of the captions on films and television (according to several researches, the deaf pass on the average 4-6 hours a day watching television), the telex news services on television, and the graphic-telephone for the deaf.

It is certainly possible to bring even multiply handicapped deaf children of normal intelligence to real reading and to at least graphic language.

Summary
In addition to deafness, two handicaps endangering an oral development in deaf children have been detected. The first is a motor handicap called apraxia or dyspraxia. A factor revealed that finger development (eupraxia), development of rhythm (eurhythmia), fluent speech, speech-reading and speech-hearing are a single factor. Apraxia or dyspraxia of the fingers and arhythmia or dysrhythmia are related to apraxia or dyspraxia of speech, including difficulty in speech-reading and speech-hearing development. However, an advantage in these children is that the memory for simultaneously presented visual data, including the graphic form of words, is typically strong. This ability can be used as a support for speech and verbal development. The second is a cognitive-motor handicap, called intermodal integration disability. The ability to read normally (eulexia) is based on the integration of the written and spoken form of words. This appears to be related to the quick use of

word meanings (eusymbolia). A disability in this intermodal integration endangers the meaningful oral functioning and the development of reading and writing. These multiple handicaps can be detected at 3 or 4 years of age. Special tests for detection of these handicaps have been developed.

I. Neurogical considerations

Literature: Benson (1979), Bok (1962), Granit (1970), Kolb and Wishaw (1980), Luchsinger and Arnold (1970), Penfield (1975), Thompson (1975), Vester (1975, 1978), Wyke (1978).

Throughout the study the following neurological theory is presupposed.

1. NEUROLOGICAL INTERCONNECTIONS

The brain contains 50,000,000 brain cells with many more interconnections. In order to appreciate the role of the brain in the present study some explanatory concepts may be helpful.

a. Stimulogeneous fibrillation and biochemical facilitation; neuro-biotaxis; synapses with stochastic functions

The terms "stimulus" and "response" or "reaction" may lead to a misunderstanding if they are taken to mean that a neurone is activated only by the influence of a stimulus. This is not the case. As long as a neurone is alive it is active and remains so, but this activity will decrease through deprivation of stimuli leading to a situation in which the neurone may even die.

"Stimulogeneous fibrillation" means that, under the influence of a stimulus, the neurone grows fibrils. Under the same influence these fibrils may lengthen in a random way, as an operant. "Stimulogeneous biochemical facilitation" means that the neurone and its fibrils undergo certain physiological changes which may facilitate the propagation of some stimuli and the inhibition of other ones in a selective and profiled way.

"Neuro-biotaxis" means that, when two brain cells are stimulated at about the same time, their fibrillations and facilitations may grow towards each other, i.e. may form a profiled pattern (see below).

"Synapses" are places of contact between neurones and their fibrils. They work selectively and in a profiled way, feeding ahead and also feeding back.

The Greek word "stochasm" literally means: guessing. The term "stochasms" can be translated by: laws of probability. The connections

19

between neurones do not work strictly determinatively, but according to laws of probability.

b. "Nature" and "nurture"
The term "nurture" may also lead to a misunderstanding, if considered only in terms of "feeding and *receiving*" food. By "nurture" we mean an ecological interaction. Every biological and psychic development must be seen as a "teamwork" of ability and ecological interaction. So neither "nurture" is onesidedly passive, nor "nature" is onesidedly active. Not only is there an interaction between the organism and its environment, but also *within* the organism an interaction of nurture and nature must be assumed.

c. Intramodal programming of parts of the brain, and "Gestalt" formations
By "intramodal" interaction is meant an interaction within the same "mode" or aspect of behaviour. By "intermodal" interaction is meant an interaction between two or more different aspects of behaviour.

"Gestalt"
It seems to be a general biological law that organisms (including cells, neurones, etc.) which start to interconnect, do so in a way of a "Gestalt". This means: selectively, profiledly, stochasticly in such a way that the whole is more than the sum of the parts.

Perceptual and motor neurones
There seems to be a developmental difference between perceptual brain cells and motor ones. The first ones seem to be more dependent on stimuli from the environment than the latter ones. Both of them atrophy by deprivation of ecological interaction, however. But one should avoid thinking of perceptual neurones in too onesided a way, as if they were purely passive. As long as they are alive, they are active, directed towards perception, "taking in", which may be described as a kind of hunger for stimuli. The motor neurones are active in another way, however, which may be described as a state of higher and lower excitation.

The "link sense"
The functions of kinesthesia, tactility and somesthesia seem to be closely connected. The perceptions of the data from skin, membranes, muscles and joints seem to lump together in one whole. Interestingly enough Stern, as early as 1935, noticed the central function of this modality, which he called the "link sense", linking all sense functions, and these sense functions with the motor system. His observation has to do with the so-called "Gerstmann syndrome".

20

"Gnosis"

"Gnosis" should be considered a special aspect of the perceptual functioning, not just knowledge or cognition in a general meaning. It is more specific, being the knowledge of an object, exemplified in figure-background discrimination, i.e. choosing a constellation within and from surrounding data. Perhaps this may be meant by the term *"re*cognition". There is gnosis happening in each modality, and also in intermodal functioning. It can be disturbed too, even when general discrimination is not disturbed. Then we speak of dysgnosia or even agnosia (see below). For example a patient may discriminate words very well, as "ball" from "bowl", but has trouble in picking out a signal in noise, in singling out a word in a discourse. This patient, suffering from an auditory figure-background discrimination disturbance, may not suffer from a visual figure-background discrimination disturbance, being able to identify a typical drawing within a series of similar drawings. Another patient may suffer from the reverse, still another patient from both disorders, etc.

The motor neurones

The motor neurones seem to be less dependent on stimuli from outside. They start spontaneously innervating muscles and joints. By doing this they may develop fibrils and biochemical facilitations. Because several motor pyramid cells are grouped within the motor brain, they may develop spontaneously at least some Gestalt formations, very much "at random" in the beginning. If they do not get a chance to actualize their innervating activities, however, e.g. by not receiving feedback from the muscles and the joints, they also will atrophy and die.

The growth, interconnections and Gestalt formations of the pyramid cells in the motor brain may be illustrated, by a kind of "model", as shown in Figure 4.

By continuous feedback from the muscles, from the joints and so from the environment, the motor brain starts to form motor Gestalts and to programme skilled movements. The programming, the Gestalt formation of a skilled movement, includes:
* the innervation of the right limbs, i.e. the finding of them;
* the co-ordination of these movements both in space and time (included sequences of movements, rhythm and planning behaviour);
* the motor memory of skills.

Eupraxia and body scheme

All of this has to do with *eupraxia*, i.e. an easy building up and maintaining of a motor programme.

It also includes a motor control of the body scheme, of left and right, of above and below, of in front of and behind, and this not only within one's

21

Figure 4.

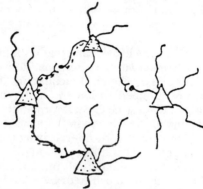

Unprogrammed brain-cells   Anatomically programmed brain-cells

Biochemically programmed brain-cells

own body, but also in the environment, by projection (e.g. "which chair is at your right side?"). See Prick and Calon (1950), Calon (1950), Prick and van der Waals (1958-1965), Prick and Calon (1967), Brown (1972).

Intransitive movements (see above)
Kaplan (1968, 1972) rightly distinguishes between so-called transitive and intransitive movements. These terms are taken from linguistics, the so-called transitive and intransitive verbs. By transitive movements are meant those movements by means of which we handle an object, e.g. moulding an object into certain shape, constructing, dressing ourselves, washing, playing tennis, etc. By intransitive movements we mean those which do not influence an object, such as dancing and speaking. (It may

22

be clear that *purely* intransitive movements are impossible: we at least move our own body.) Intransitive movements need more eupraxia than transitive ones, because these latter ones have a clear feedback from the object: the object helps to control the movements, to find the right "steering".

It may be clear from this that the eupraxia-dyspraxia-apraxia of a person are investigated more clearly and deeply by using tests of intransitive movements. We will explain below how we have applied this principle in our research.

Gestalt formation and autonomy
Where there is Gestalt formation, there is also autonomy. It is the law of a Gestalt that it "strives" after the maintenance and expansion of itself.

All of us have visual Gestalts in our mind, which proceed to images, fantasy and to memory; figure-background functioning is involved too. It is the same with auditory Gestalts, tactual Gestalts, olfactory and gustatory Gestalts, kinesthetic Gestalts, motor Gestalts. All these Gestalts maintain a certain independency towards each other, although they also are closely interconnected. Furthermore: all these Gestalt formations include a certain hierarchy of sub-Gestalts, embedded and embracing Gestalts, etc.

Lashley (1951) tried to prove the autonomy of a motor programming, by emphasizing the phenomenon of very rapid movements: he thought the reaction-time from the sensory motor control may be too short for a "point to point monitoring". Perhaps the speed of sensory information is high enough, but with regard to the complexity of many movements, he may be right.

d. Normal distributions of functions
Many, if not all functions of nature show a so-called normal distribution, i.e. about 16% of the subordinates are "high", 68% "moderate" and 16% "low" in a specific function. Intelligence seems to be normally distributed: there are persons of high intelligence, moderate intelligence and below moderate intelligence. The same with muscular strength, etc. In our very demanding society it is possible that a function, although within the range of moderate strength, but below the average, is already showing an impairment.

These same normal distributions are found in the functions of perception, perhaps not so much in their primary function, but certainly in the so-called associative and apperceptional functions. This is shown by very many tests, e.g. for the visual and auditory function: figure-background formation, speed of learning, memory, etc.

The same must be said about motor programming. Again the same may be said about intramodal integration, intermodal integration, etc.

A tripartite terminology

In many studies a tripartite terminology is used, e.g. eurhythmia, dys-rhythmia and arhythmia (cf. Fraisse, 1956, 1974). Meaning a good rhythmic behaviour, a disturbed rhythmic behaviour and the absence or almost absence of rhythmic behaviour. Dys- means disturbed, a- means absent or lacking. In the same way we may speak of:

eupraxia, dyspraxia and apraxia (the term "eupraxia" was first used by Cobb, 1948);
euphasia, dysphasia and aphasia;
eulexia, dyslexia and alexia;
eugraphia, dysgraphia and agraphia;
eugnosia, dysgnosia and agnosia;
eusymbolia, dyssymbolia and asymbolia;
eucalculia, dyscalculia and acalculia.

Weaknesses in one function can be *compensated* by strength in another function. For example, a normal hearing person may suffer from dys-praxia, but this dyspraxia may not turn into dyspraxia of speech, a kind of dysphasia, because he can compensate by a very strong auditory per-ception and memory. But a similar dyspraxia in a deaf person may turn into a dyspraxia of speech and dysphasia, because he cannot compen-sate.

Innate abilities, disabilities?

It seems to be incorrect to attribute the normal distribution of a function *only* to ecological interaction. An innate ability must be assumed. There certainly is an innate high ability in some persons, a moderate innate ability in the vast majority and again a low innate ability in some persons. So we must speak of "rich and poor brain fields", which may be illustra-ted just by a kind of "model", in this way (Figure 5).

e. Intermodal integration and "governing" of behaviour

We now speak of the interconnections between brain fields.

"Governing" means steering, ruling. The Greek term *"cybernetics"* has been chosen by Wiener (1947, see van Uden, 1962) for the science of steering functions in culture and nature (physics, biology, physiology, psychology, sociology, economics, etc.). This Greek word is the root of the English word governing (cybern = govern).

By "steering", "governing" is meant here: the reciprocal influence of neurones, with feeding ahead and feeding back processes (= cybernetic processes), for both an internal and an external adaptation, assimilation and direction. It must be said that each Gestalt formation includes cybernetic processes, both intra a brainfield and inter brainfields.

24

Figure 5

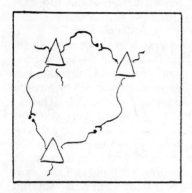

A poor motor programming
field in the brain.

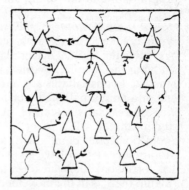

A rich motor programming
field in the brain.

The poverty of the motor field in the brain has been drawn here in an anatomic way, but it can and must be conceived also in a biochemical way. Many studies have shown that several functions of man are hereditary, not only the riches of innate ability but also its poverty. But such as poverty or weakness can originate from illnesses too, from infections (e.g. rubella), atrophies, a shock, a hemorrhage, enlarged ventricles, etc.

"Steering from point to point"
Let us take an example from the driving of a car. If we start to do so, our motor functions, more precisely our *ef*ferent functions, our conative functions, are first: "We *want* to drive a car" (see below). While driving our car, our movements are followed by our eyes from point to point; they are corrected, brought to a successful end. We must be aware, many motoric Gestalts are working *within* that steering process. These are not followed by the eyes from point to point, but are released by a firing *trigger* "as of an automatic gun", more or less autonomous, running automatically. Besides, this steering by the eyes should not be conceived of as only a conscious process: an expert car driver will mainly drive his car automatically; he may be able to have long and intense conversations while driving. But the same expert car driver will react, not only when a mistaken movement has actually appeared, but even before, in a *anticipatory* way, as soon as there appears something *threatening* in his movements.
It must be emphasized that the *"triggering effect"* mentioned above is

25

not only working for a motor programming, but for all other kinds of programming in our brain, and for the perceptual programs too.

How a sensory motor Gestalt steering process is developing
We may take as an example learning to declutch in car driving. In the beginning the student driver may learn it in a verbal way, by reading and studying the manual, by memorizing it and putting the direction into practice. Let us call this a "considering function", which can be a verbal one or a nonverbal one by means of a diagram, a gesture, etc. This is a kind of associative steering, mainly point to point. But very soon our student driver will go over to a kind of rhythmic guidance, by saying: "pom pom-pom pom". Several researches (e.g. van der Veldt, 1928, Montpellier, 1935) have shown that tempo and rhythm of movements are correlated: the quicker a tempo, the more rhythm; and the more rhythm there is in the movement, the quicker tempo can grow. Rhythm and tempo can increase in such a way that an autonomous sensori-motoric Gestaltformation originates. The tactual stimulus, e.g. by grasping the clutch, may "trigger" that programme. This embracing sensori-motor Gestaltformation may include sub-Gestalts, namely the Gestalt of the motor brain, the kinesthetic-tactile Gestalt, perhaps also the auditory Gestalt (the sound of the engine), etc.

It must be emphasized again that the automatic "going off" of these programmes does not prevent an *anticipatory* steering.

It may be clear that the more difficult the movement, the more time and training will be necessary to learn it. See how a ballet dancer trains: he deliberates his movements, feels them, uses music mainly to make them as rhythmic as possible, uses a mirror, etc. The same must be said about the learning to speak by a deaf child, more so if the child has a dyspraxia.

Here we see how a strong auditory function, with a strong auditory memory, may *compensate* the dyspraxia in many persons. When a new word has to be learned, especially when the pronunciation is rather difficult, such a person may try to hear the word in a slower tempo, to articulate it in a more pronounced fashion, to look at its written form, etc. We also know that not all normal hearing children learn to speak at the same age, and this not only because of the environment, but also because of their degree of auditory memory, degree of eupraxia, etc.

All of this concerns the steering, and sometimes also the compensating function of our brain from the sensory field towards the motoric field. But there are reciprocal influences between the sensory fields too, e.g. between the auditory and the visual fields, resulting in both auditory and visual profiles of perception, imagination and memory.

Therefore, it can not be said that Gestalt formation, programming will no longer be possible, when a special field of the brain is poor or weak.

26

This can only be said when that poverty would have been reduced to nothing or almost nothing. But even a poor field is "Gestaltable", "programmable", to a certain extent.

Loop processes and constants
How do the processes of adaptation, assimilation, adjustment of the organism to the environment develop? Here we have to mention the loop processes and the constants:

The line of this development seems to include: from self-imitation towards the imitation of others, from adjustment to self towards adjustment to others. Two examples seem to be very striking: the development of grasping, and the development of speech.

The development of *grasping*. – After the first, mainly reflex-like gripping reactions, including the Moro reflex, a typical behaviour appears: a baby of about 2 months of age "examines" his own hand and finger movements, which precedes and introduces grasping of objects, improving it more and more (Piaget, 1923; Werner H., 1928; Bayley, 1935; Gesell, 1940; Prick and Calon, 1950). White, Castle and Held (1964) stated more precisely how a baby at about 0;4 years of age looks alternatively at his own hand and at the object to be handled, as if he compares them; they further found that children of a residential institution stuck to this behaviour for too long a time, which delay could be corrected by stimulation, however (White and Held, 1966).

The development of *babbling* in relation to speaking seems to be analogous to the development of grasping. The first babbling seems to be a kind of self-imitation of the baby, comparable with the looking at the movements of his own hand and fingers, described above. He not only imitates his articulatory sounding movements, but also his melodies (cf. Weir, 1962). At the same time speech and melodies from the environment, especially from the mother, are instilled into the loop processes of his melodious babbling, as constants, comparable with the objects to be grasped and to be adjusted to. From about 0;6-0;8 months of age echolalic babbling appears, together with the three intonations of question, assertion and call or appeal ("emphatic intonation", Menyuk, 1969). More and more the organism of the baby adjusts itself to the speech and the melodies of the environment.

Gibson (1958, cit. Kohler, 1966) broadens the concept "proprio-ception" towards "proprio-re-ception", perhaps better called "proprio-*per*-ception". At the moment we hear our own movements of arms and legs and body and mouth, see ourselves, touch and handle our body, etc., these proprio-per-ceptions, the proprio-*cep*tion and the motor programmings are pushed together into one whole, one pattern, one "Gestalt". This seems to be a necessary preparation of and introduction to a coordinated handling of an object and to a more and more correct imitating of others.

27

The first loop processes are, relatively speaking, rather variable, flexible and plastic, in comparison to the developing automated skills, adjusted to the constants from the environment. We conclude that it is not the stimulus-response which is the basic model of behaviour, but the "motus sui", life itself, the "operant" according to the terminology of Skinner (1957). This development can be illustrated by the following diagram:

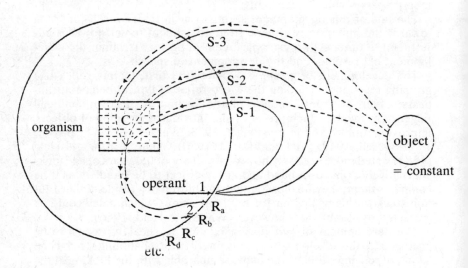

Explanation:
(1) It starts with the operant = spontaneous motor behaviour.
   S-1, S-2, S-3 = proprio-ception and proprio-per-ception.
   C = comparator; the spontaneous motoric-sensoric behaviour is stereotyped and profiled; the comparator works as a norm.
(2) R_a = reaction or response; the operant develops towards modified, more determined forms of reaction, guided by the comparator.
Object = a constant, working upon the organism from outside; it may be evoked by the organism itself, but very often it is not. An example of such a constant, such a "object" is the speech of the mother towards her babbling child. These stimuli from outside are integrated into the loop processes. In this way the reactions develop towards R_b, and further towards R_c etc. = towards sensori-motoric skills.
   All these processes must be seen as "aiming at" an integrated unity of the organism.

28

For further explanation of this development see Tatham (1980, see Moore, 1981): the initial state of the development is a random activity, with subsequent learning of constraints.

Strong, moderate and weak integration
The intermodal integration function seems to be normally distributed. For example, Koppitz (1972) found that the integration of a heard series of digits with its written form and vice versa is normally distributed among children. Whitacker and Noll (1972) found the same for the integration of heard words and their meanings.

We will find children and adults having a very strong intermodal integration function, others having only a moderate one, and still others being weak and very weak in this function. We have met some of those patients, suffering from integration dyslexia or alexia, dyssymbolia or even asymbolia: all of these patients need a very individual treatment.

The strength of a chain is dependent on the strength of each link
It seems to be clear that, if one element of the intermodal constellation is missing or functioning very weakly, the intermodal integration as a whole will be endangered. A few examples:
   Children born blind show some typical speech defects (see below), in the beginning. The integration of the speech sounds heard from the mother, from whom they cannot see the articulation, does not integrate with their own articulation quickly enough. – A sentence read in Braille integrates less quickly as a tactual whole than a sentence read by seeing (Révèsz, 1938).
   Prelingually deaf children, mainly depending on lipreading, have more difficulty in integrating the written form of a word and its spoken form. A normally hearing child may see the written form and hear its spoken form, synchronically. Not so a deaf child: at the moment he sees the written form by reading, he cannot see its spoken form by lipreading. For the same reason the experience of a flower may integrate less easily with its spoken lipread form. A normally hearing child hears the word while e.g. picking and seeing the flower. A deaf child has to look up at his mother in order to lipread the word flower, and at that moment does not see the flower. The integration of the experiences with the words is endangered more in deaf children than in normally hearing children, i.e. endangered by "verbiage" (empty words) and dyssymbolia.
   An effect of this situation will be that, if a "full sensed" child has some weakness in its intermodal integration function, he will be less endangered than a "less sensed" child. The latter children will develop dyslexia and dyssymbolia more easily.
   Dyspraxia shows an analogous phenomenon. It will result in dysphasia

in hearing impaired children and children with a weak auditory memory, more so than in normally hearing children (see below). One also sees a typical phenomenon in dyspraxic or apraxic children and adults in their way of drawing and writing. Especially young dyspraxic children may draw in very short stripes or strokes or lines. The reason is obvious: they have less ability to monitor their drawing by their motor programming, and are more dependent on seeing to compensate, i.e. on monitoring afterwards. When a eupraxic person draws with a pencil, he "feels", *while* moving, his hand, whether his movement is correct or not, anticipatorily and synchronously. How can a dyspraxic one, having a difficulty in programming his movements, know whether his line is correct or not? Only be seeing it, i.e. a little bit afterwards. If he draws quickly, he almost always does so by an insufficiently prepared movement: he may make a mistake (e.g. too long a line, not in the correct direction, etc.). He will try to avoid that and starts to draw in short stripes, looking at the visible effects again and again. So he compensates for his clumsiness and gets a good line (Figure 6).

Figure 6.

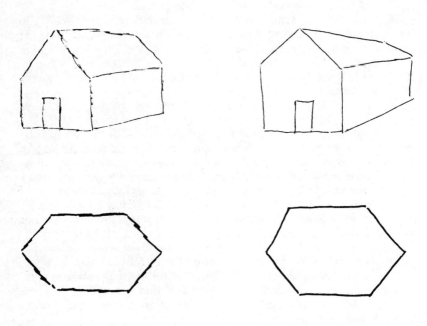

Drawings by a dyspraxic child.   Drawings by a eupraxic child.

Another way of compensation is to draw or write very very slowly.

Cortical and subcortical functions; two hemispheres of the brain
The intermodal integration should not be thought of as if it were only cortical and in one hemisphere of the brain. Obviously it has to do with subcortical processes too, with the interaction of cortical and subcortical processes and, last but not least, with the interaction between the two hemispheres, always in "Gestalt forming" ways.

Summary
The development and functioning of neurological Gestalt formations are described. Emphasis is put on motor programming, the control of the body scheme and on cybernetic functions. Intramodal and intermodal integrations are described. Innate functiones can be strong, moderate or weak.

2. THE EFFERENCE PRINCIPLE. BODY SCHEME. MEMORY

a. The efference principle
"Efference" contrasts with "afference". The efference means all the reactions of the organism towards the environment. The afference means all the stimuli received in the organism from the environment.

The efference principle means that all the responses, the (re-)actions, have to be seen as one whole, as one hierarchic Gestalt, comprising sub-Gestalts, and that this efference has a strong influence on the afference, according to the old adagium: "Quidquid recipitur ad modum recipientis recipitur", i.e. whatever is received, is received in the way of the (active) receiver.

Thus the efference integrates with the afference in interaction.

The efference comprises motor functions (do not forget the expressive motor functions, both oral-verbal and non-verbal), motivation, emotion and conation. Motivation has a strong integrating power on the whole of the behaviour of the organism. Think of the so-called "orienting reflex" and the concentration. Lack of motivation has desintegrating effects on behaviour. For this reason it is not so easy to diagnose an authentic intermodal integration disturbance: it may happen that a child is reacting very desintegratedly, showing dyslexia and dyssymbolia, just by lack of motivation. If that same child becomes more motivated afterwards, all effects of desintegration may disappear.

The challenging of the afference
A perception will not develop or will develop only weakly, unless its function is challenged. The environment must challenge the perception,

i.e. evoke motivation. If not, the perceptual function will not come to its full potential. This is one of the strongest influences from the efference towards the afference. A few examples:

For example, a normally hearing child of 7 years in the elementary school has already learned to read well technically, but becomes more and more visually handicapped. One has tried to teach the child *Braille*. But he never learns Braille as long as he can see the letters. If he becomes blind, a situation in which he would no longer be able to see letters, he could possibly learn Braille within a few weeks. The reason is obvious: in the latter situation his tactual sense is challenged, in the first one it is not. – Blind people may develop a very strong memory of the *voices* and way of speaking of other people, much better than normally seeing people do. They may recognize and identify a voice after years! The reason is that this hearing function is challenged. – A farmer knows by name his *100 cows*, but an outsider does not even see big differences between them. – An expert car-driver or cyclist notices each cue on the *road* while his companion, not having that skill, "sees nothing".

Another example is *lipreading*: this function will not develop unless it is challenged by the oral environment. An important remark: if a school for the deaf is following a spontaneous conversational method of teaching language, the lipreading function of its children will become on the average very strong. Not so, if a school is following a programmed way of teaching language, lacking spontaneous conversation. In the latter situation the words, the sentences become highly predictable: the child may know in advance which word or which sentence will be presented to him to be lipread. The lipreading function of the children is not challenged enough and will not develop to its full potential. Interestingly enough a call for "supporting signs", "fingerspellling", "Cued Speech" (Cornett, 1967) is heard in the latter schools, not in the first ones. The reason is obvious: spontaneous conversation always strongly challenges the lipreading function. By that same continuous challenge and motivation hard-of-hearing children and adults, tested by means of a silent lipreading film, appear to have learned lipreading themselves without formal training, even significantly better than prelingually and postlingually profoundly deaf children and adults (see O'Neill, 1961; Berger, 1972; Oyer et al., 1975). The reason seems to be obvious: they experience every day how their understanding is improved by watching the speaker, which improvement reinforces that function; in addition to this they have on the average much more spontaneous conversations than the deaf.

The same must be said about the *auditory* function (Oyer, 1966). Deaf children (cf. Markides, 1976) and adults (cf. Higgins, 1980), in "manual" settings (i.e. mainly using and emphasizing sign codes for the daily conversations), usually develop their auditory function insufficiently, may even reject the hearing aid, in contrast to deaf people, whose hearing is continuously challenged and who are motivated to use it.

b. The body scheme
The term "body scheme" has to do both with the "gross limbs" (e.g. arms and legs) and with the "fine limbs" (e.g. the articulators for speech). Literally speaking the term means the distribution of the limbs of the body in space: right, middle, left – above, middle, below – in front of, middle, behind – left above, middle, right below etc.

Most important is the "body scheme control". This comprises the following aspects:

The motor control, in the sense of motor eupraxia in the motor fields of the brain.

The sensory control (kinesthetic tactual, somesthetic, visual, auditory etc.), again by means of Gestalt formation both of the perceptual fields and of the intermodal integration. Prick and Calon (1950) speak of "body-relation-recognition".

This control means: the quick finding of the right limbs and their coordination, so that a specific action can be executed correctly. By means of projection the control of the body scheme originates a control of space, e.g. what do you see above, below, in front of, behind, right or left? See above. (Remlein-Mozalewska (1980) seems to have forgotten the link between body scheme control and its projection in space control.)

c. The memory function (van Uden, 1980, 1981)
This again is a very complex concept, which we can analyse in four aspects:
- The cognitive intramodal memory, i.e. not only on the basis of sensory imput, but also of fantasy (e.g. the memory of a dream). It is found in all modalities. The function is not always as strong in all modalities: people may show a typical memory profile, e.g. being strong in auditory memory but weak in visual memory etc.
- Cognitive intermodal memory, e.g. by means of associative functions.
- Conative memory: e.g. an old forgotten want may spontaneously reappear.
- Motor memory: e.g. we have not ridden a bicycle for years and notwithstanding that we may experience that we have not forgotten that skill, at the moment we unexpectedly have to ride again.

"Memory" in a more general sense can be described as: "retrieval function".

Summary
The interaction of efferent and afferent behaviour is explained, emphasizing the necessity of challenging the afferent functions for a devel-

opment to their full potential. Also the control of the body scheme develops by interaction. All of this converges into four aspects of the memory function.

3. DESCRIPTION OF SOME DISTURBANCES AND DISABILITIES

Aphasia, alexia, agraphia, acalculia, asymbolia etc. are terms used by neurologists almost exclusively as *a loss* of the functions meant by these words. In the last 50 years we see the appearance of the term "developmental aphasia" (e.g. Ewing "Aphasia in children", 1930), "developmental alexia" etc., not as a loss in the same sense, but as a handicap in the development, by some innate malfunction or by an acquired damage in the early months of life.

Dysphasia and even aphasia may originate from a motor dyspraxia and apraxia and/or from an intermodal integration disturbance.

Dysarthria and anarthria are regarded in this book as speech disturbances, originating from difficulties with the tactual sense in the mouth and/or malfunctions in the extra-pyramidal subcortical centres, via choreo-athetosis, choreo-formity, athetoidia etc. Sometimes these disturbances may be so small that only a very accurate and intensive observation may discover them.

Perceptual disturbances.
There are several disturbances to be found in the auditory and/or visual behaviour, apart from threshold-losses, especially in the functions of:
- discrimination,
- processing, particularly slowness, originating overlappings of inputs and similar; e.g. a patient suffering from bradyacousia, hearing a phrase like "happily enough", spoken at a normal tempo, may perceive the beginning of "enough", while the sound of "happily" is not yet processed in his mind, so that both words become confused and not understood; another patient, suffering from an analogous disturbance in the visual mode of perception, may see some objects or pictures or words overlapping, originating confusions, e.g. in reading (bradylexia, a kind of perceptual dyslexia), etc.,
- figure-background perception (gnosis); e.g. a patient may be able to copy a figure like:

but may get into trouble, if he has to identify the right figure in a series:

34

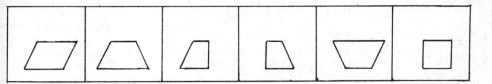

This disturbance may originate another kind of perceptual dyslexia, and also dysgraphia (cf. Satz and Nostrand, 1973; Callaway, 1975; Wissen and Biesalski, 1977; Gross and Rothenberg, 1979).
- memory, both short-term memory and long-term memory.
- difficulties with the tactual sense in the mouth, i.e. the "tactile oral stereognosis", see Ringel and Steer (1963), Ringel, House, Buck, Dolinski and Scott (1970), Edwards (1970), Locke (1969), Scott and Ringel (1971), Gammon a.o. (1971), Bishop, Ringel and House (1972).
These difficulties will not be studied here.

Dysgraphia and agraphia should be described very carefully:
- A child may write a word completely different from what he had spoken: e.g. he spoke Mary and if asked to write it down, he may write "John". The reason may be a very strong intermodal integration problem, a kind of graphic word finding disturbance.
- It may happen that a young deaf child does not start to write: he does not imitate by drawing and the function of writing does not develop. The pocket typewriter "Communicator" (Canon Manufactories) is very often a godsend: the child starts to typewrite the word and by means of this he starts writing.
- A child may produce many writing errors, so often that it is a real disturbance, a dysgraphia. For example, he may speak ball correctly but write bad or dab; – he may speak warm but write marv or mraw.....
This third phenomenon is the most common one, and can have different causes:
- A child, suffering from dyspraxia or apraxia, will have difficulty in discriminating e.g. d and b. The difficulty is a projective one, originating from his disturbed control of the body scheme. He can only conquer the difficulty by a very strong visual perception and memory. But by a combination of dyspraxia-apraxia and weak visual memory a primary dysgraphia will arise, an original and a very difficult disability.
- Another cause, happily enough not a very common one, is a weak figure-background discrimination, by which confusions arise as
n = m = w;
b = 1 = k; *b = l = k;*

o = a; o ≠ a
e = c;
eu = oe etc.

The longer a word the more disturbance will be felt. This is another kind of primary dysgraphia.

- There is also a secondary dysgraphia, however. This is the effect of a wrong treatment or of the neglect of a treatment. For example, a teacher may train a child suffering from dyspraxia and/or from an intermodal integration disturbance, in writing while speaking, or speaking while writing, in order to promote a strong integration of both functions. This is a good training method indeed, provided the child does not have the learning disabilities mentioned just now. Very often the effect now is very bad writing. The reason is obvious: because of his learning disability the child is not giving attention enough to the written form of the word. Because of this he does not imprint that written form, and because of this again he simply forgets. These kind of children need, first of all, a *direct* imprinting of the written form of the words, without speaking, e.g. by using a typewriter or the Communicator (Canon).

– The integration of the written and the spoken form should not be forgotten, however: as soon as the child is able both to write some words from memory, and to speak them by heart, the integration of *these* words must be trained, together with a strong phonetic and graphic analysis. An example: suppose such a child is able to speak "cupboard", but is not able yet to write (or type) this word from memory, we have to postpone the integration of the spoken and the written form of *this* word. We first look for other words, both spoken from memory and written from memory, e.g. ball, car, table, bed. We teach the term *vowel*, because the vowels have the most various spellings:

"Look for the *vowel:* a – e and the *vowel-symbols*!"

"Find the *b* and pronounce it! Find the *l* ", etc.

See the "Northampton Vowel and Consonant cards" (Clarke School, 1972).

Dyslexia and alexia: this disturbance parallels the dysgraphia-agraphia

36

mentioned above. There are two kinds of primary dyslexia-alexia:
- integrative dyslexia-alexia, which includes that the spoken and the written forms of words integrate only difficultly, together with a difficult integration of the symbol (word) and its meaning (dyssymbolia-asymbolia), both originating from an intermodal integration disturbance;
- perceptual dyslexia-alexia on account of a visual figure-background disturbance.

Dyscalculia and acalculia
The deepest form of this disturbance is that the child does not see quantities quickly enough: "Are there three, seven, four beads?" etc. This disturbance seldom happens. Another, less deep but more frequent difficulty concerns quantitative relations and proportions, e.g. in lines, contours, perspective and in digits: "How many more apples are there?" "How many cubes are in the horizontal line in front of the vertical line?" etc. Another difficulty is that of finding the right mathematical operation or series of operations: addition, subtraction, multiplication, division.

Usually dyscalculia-acalculia is caused by a combination of dyspraxia-apraxia and sensori-motor integration disturbance (usually including dyslexia-alexia). On account of dyspraxia-apraxia the child does not see spatial relations, constellations and quantities in the right way, by a projection of his body scheme disturbance. On account of the sensory motor integration disturbance the child does not understand or find the symbols with their meanings. One sees the difficulty arising even in the nursery school. Observe some children when they are counting on their fingers: two fingers over each other, repeating the same finger etc., with the effect that the resulting figure is wrong. One sees that this child simply cannot find his fingers, neither motorily, nor visually, nor tactually.

Sometimes it happens that a child developing dyscalculia is not developing dyslexia: the reason usually is that the child is highly intelligent, living in a very rich and varied environment with much conversation. By means of this the child has learned to interpret a written text correctly from a few visual cues. But in calculation and mathematics he makes a clean breast of his deep disturbance.

Summary
The most common learning disabilities in deaf children are described: aphasia, dysarthria, perceptual disturbances, dysgraphia, dyslexia and dyscalculia.

4. TREATMENT BY SWITCHING ON COMPENSATORY FUNCTIONS

The main aim of rehabilitation should be seen in terms of a diagnosis of the strong abilities of the child, of developing them and of integrating them into the child's whole behaviour pattern, thus of using compensatory functions.

For example, dyspraxic children very often show a strong visual memory for simultaneously presented data (see chapter V and VI). These children can develop a strong memory for the written form of the words, which in its turn becomes a support for their speech. Furthermore their creativity and spontaneity should be used, for developing rhythmics, planning behaviour, steering behaviour. Because the motor functions are primary, all training should be active and one-sided passivity should be avoided. Important activities should be verbalized, in order to originate transfer and intermodal integration, e.g. by analysing situations, figures and constellations and by describing such an analysis verbally.

II. Development of eupraxia of speech, i.e. of speech programming in the brain, in congenitally profoundly deaf children

1. BABBLING, *NOT INFLUENCED YET* BY THE WEARING OF A HEARING AID, NOR BY A "CONSTANT" FROM OUTSIDE

a. Use of voice and babbling

Lenneberg (1967) found that the *voice* of a very young deaf child is completely normal when he is relaxed, e.g. when laughing. The opposite happens when he is under stress (Jacobs, 1968; Löwe, 1970).

Mowrer (1950), Myklebust (1957) and Mindel and Vernon (1971) deny that congenitally profoundly deaf babies *babble*. These assertions are not in agreement with scientifically controlled evidence. I myself observed a congenitally profoundly deaf boy of 1;2 years of age and noted e.g.: "gogowa ... wodoh ... ahwohwah ..." for almost 8 seconds. We quote Nanninga-Boon (1929), Kampik (1930), Rau (1935), Gloyer (1961, cf. Paziner, 1966, report about twins, of which one was normally hearing, the other one profoundly deaf), Köble (1962, a rubella deaf child), Lenneberg et al. (1965, babies of congenitally deaf parents, one baby being profoundly deaf), Mavilya (1969, 1970).

Summarizing the data: in the beginning the babbling of congenitally profoundly deaf children is not qualitatively different from that of normally hearing children. But quantitatively there are differences. On the average, profoundly deaf children babble much less than normally hearing children, and the percentage of the observation time decreases constantly, so that, at about 6-7 months of age, it does not comprise more than a few minutes of an hour's observation time. There is also less self-imitation and more dominance of vowels over consonants than in normally hearing babies. Nothing has been found which could be considered a kind of intonation, but there are rhythmic iterations, although shorter than in normally hearing babies. The lengths of the "breath-units" (a term of Irwin's, 1947) comprise on the average only three phonemes per unit.

After about 0;6 months the babbling deteriorates more and more, although it almost never stops completely. See below.

b. The *similarity* between the babbling of congenitally profoundly deaf babies and that of normally hearing babies
This may be illustrated as follows:

The average relative frequencies of the vowels of deaf babies aged from 0;3 to 0;6 months (data by Mavilya, 1969) have been converted into percentages of the total in order to compare them with the frequencies of normally hearing babies aged 0;3 to 0;4 and 0;5 to 0;6 months according to Chen (1946) and Irwin (1947). There are 8 American-English vowels involved. The data of the deaf babies are correlated with those of Chen's normally hearing babies .71 (product moment correlation $p < 0.05$) and with the data according to Irwin .73 ($p < 0.05$).

We conclude that loop processes of speech exist in profoundly deaf babies, although much less than in normally hearing ones. These processes work not according to an auditory or a visual loop, but solely to an articulatory one, which definitely has an effect but clearly less strongly. As long as there is no influence from outside, i.e. no "constant", the growth will be very very poor. Lach et al. (1970) investigated the babbling of deaf babies, about 1 year older than those mentioned above (0;11-2;9 years of age). One of these babies was profoundly deaf (100 dB). Where the vowels are concerned, there is no difference between this and the data of Mavilya (1969) of deaf babies of 0;6 months of age. There were a few more consonants, the relative frequencies of which are similar to those of a normally hearing baby of 0;6 months of age (Irwin, 1947). The data by Sykes (1940) of deaf infants 3;10 to 6;10 years of age, 8 of whom were prelingually profoundly deaf, show again a growth of consonants, from 11% at Lach's investigation to 32%. The children babbled and vocalized only $1/2$% of the observation time, however. Carr (1953) investigated the spontaneous babbling and vocalizations of 48 prelingually deaf children of 5 years of age. She found 41% consonants. The "breath-units" comprised on the average 4 phonemes. (Also these children were not yet wearing a hearing aid.) It is possible to calculate "product-moment correlations" between her data and those of normally hearing children (Irwin, 1947, 1948), see Table 3.

The deterioration of the frequency of vowel utterances is clear. The profiles of the consonants show a small improvement.

We compared Sykes' data (1940) with those of Carr (1953) and we found a product-moment correlation of .82 ($p < 0.01$) for the consonants, and of .50 (not significant) for the vowels. The data of these two studies seem to be reliable.

40

Table 3.

Frequency profile of	Correlations of the frequency profiles of deaf children of 5 years of age with those of the following *hearing* children		
	of 0;6 years of age	of 1;0 years of age	of 2;0 years of age
Vowels	.84**	.90**	.13
Consonants	.46*	.52**	.57**

* = p < 0.05   ** = p < 0.01

c. Babbling of deaf babies and normal *eupraxia* of speech

The articulatory loop, working in deaf children, seems to apply as well in normally hearing children. It is known that the correct pronunciation of the consonants, i.e. the eupraxia of consonants, develops in normally hearing children more slowly than that of vowels. While the eupraxia of vowels is correct usually at 3 years of age, that of the consonants occurs only at 8 years of age. The data of Menyuk (1969) show the order in which a normally hearing child learns the eupraxia of the consonants. We (van Uden, 1974) calculated rank-correlations of the frequency profiles of consonants in deaf children with this order of eupraxia. Sykes' data show a correlation of .73 (p < 0.01) and those of Carr .79 (p < 0.01). Deaf children babble those consonants most frequently which are pronounced by normally hearing children first.

The data of Lach and others, Sykes and Carr have been confirmed by those of the "Kansas Studies" under the guidance of J. Miller, the studies of Neas (1953), McCarty (1954), Houchins (1954) and Fort (1955)*.

2. IS THE EUPRAXIA OF SPEECH IN DEAF BABIES (I.E. THE DEVELOPMENT OF SPEECH PROGRAMMING IN THE BRAIN) *INFLUENCED* BY A "CONSTANT" FROM OUTSIDE?

a. "Face-directedness", use of voice, lipreading and reaction to hearing aid

Two factors seem to be very important: the habit of watching the face ("face directedness"), which may develop into lipreading, and the use of sound perception through hearing aids.

---

* These children of 70 dB and more hearing losses were not yet wearing a hearing aid. No factors had been found linking hearing loss, intelligence, time at preschool, socio-economic status of the parents, attitude of parents, difference of situations. It was noted, however, that in team games the variety of vowels and consonants increased.

41

The following survey study may illustrate the case (van Uden, 1959).

Face-directedness, use of voice, vocalisation and babbling, lipreading ability and reaction to the hearing aid have been investigated in 72 congenitally profoundly deaf children aged 0;6-5;7 years. These children were randomly selected from the data of our hometraining service, headed by Mrs. L. Bogaartz-van Uden, in the years 1955 to 1958. The ages at commencement varied from 0;6 to 5;4 years. The treatment extended from commencement to admission into the nursery school for the deaf, at the age of 4 years or older. Sometimes the time of treatment comprised $2^{1}/_{2}$ years, sometimes only a few months. Reports were made out regularly and each child was discussed individually at staff-meetings during which the following typification was given by the experienced instructresses:

face-directedness: strong or weak;
spontaneous use of voice: much or little;
lipreading ability after some time of treatment: strong or weak;
reaction to hearing aid: clear or unclear.

(1) Connection between face-directedness and age at commencement (Table 4).

Table 4.

Age at commencement	Number of children	Percentage of children who are strongly face-directed
0;6-1;12	11	8 = 72%
2;0-2;12	23	12 = 52%
3;0-3;12	20	5 = 25%
4;0-4;12	11	3 = 27%
5;0-5;4	7	1 = 14%

χ^2 16.111 df. 4 p < 0.01

Age of commencement means that before that age, there was no real treatment at all. We see a strong relation: the later the treatment started, the smaller the number of children who were strongly face-directed. Further there is a clear break after about $2^{1}/_{2}$ years of age, which will be discussed below.

(2) Connection between spontaneous use of voice and age at commencement (Table 5).

Table 5.

Age at commencement	Number of children	Percentage of children with much voice usage
0;6-1;12	11	7 = 64%
2;0-2;12	23	18 = 79%
3;0-3;12	20	13 − 64%
4;0-4;12	11	5 = 46%
5;0-5;4	7	2 = 43%

The data grouped into a 2 x 2 table of younger and older children, and of much and little voice usage:
χ^2 3.343 df. 1 p = 0.07

We see a tendency: the older the age at commencement the less voice usage.

(3) Connection between face-directedness and use of voice (Table 6).

Table 6.

Face-directedness	Use of voice		
	little	much	total
1. Maintained	6	25	31
2. Lost but regained:	2	27	29
3. Lost and not yet regained	8	4	12
χ^2 17.853 df. 2 p < 0.05.			72

(4) Connection between face-directedness and lipreading ability (Table 7).

Table 7.

Face-directedness	Lipreading ability		
	weak	strong	total
1. Maintained	5	26	31
2. Lost but regained	13	16	29
χ^2 4.59 df. 1 p < 0.05			60

Twelve children had not yet regained their face-directedness at the time of the investigation, see Table 6.

(5) Connection between face-directedness and reaction to hearing aid (Table 8).

Table 8.

Face-directedness	Reaction to hearing aid		
	unclear	clear	total
1. Maintained	8	23	31
2. Lost but regained	9	20	29
3. Lost and not yet regained	9	3	12
χ^2 9.6 df. 2 p < 0.01			72

(6) Connection between use of voice and reaction to hearing aid (Table 9).

Table 9.

Use of voice	Reaction to hearing aid		
	unclear	clear	total
Little	12	4	16
Much	14	42	56
χ^2 13.516 df. 1 p < 0.01			72

We have seen that, where the commencement started before 1;6 years of age, the majority of deaf children had a strong *face-directedness,* the same as in normally hearing children. After that age more and more children were found to have lost that face-directedness. This means that those children had become more and more directed towards the small space between their hands and eyes. It was more difficult to catch their gaze. Ewing and Ewing (1943, 1971) explained this phenomenon by the fact that most of these children at that age start to crawl and walk. Before that time, they were mainly lying on their back, naturally directed towards the face of their mother or caretaker. While a normally hearing child keeps his contact with the mother by his hearing, deaf children lose

44

it. They may become more and more "egocentric", sometimes even with traits of an atypical "autistiform" behaviour.

b. "Face-directedness" maintained or regained

How can *face-directedness* be *maintained,* and, if lost, *regained*? J. Miller (1970) has shown how the kind face of the mother or caretaker works as a reward upon an operant: they were taught to speak kindly to their child of about $1^1/_2$ years of age, as soon as it looked towards her face. The eye contact increased from on the average 1.3 per minute to 5.6 per minute. After all each child likes the face of his mother. Such behaviour has to do with acceptance processes too. Greenstein (1975) has shown that the frequency of eye contact is significantly correlated both with the amount of acceptance behaviour and the growth of language. This last aspect includes both lipreading and listening to the voice of the mother, i.e., mother's speech becomes the constant influencing the eupraxia of babbling, guiding it towards speech. Ewing and Ewing (1943, 1971) have shown how lipreading evokes speech. Downs (1968) investigated a prelingually profoundly deaf child in a longitudinal way from 0;4 to 1;2 years of age. The babbling of the child was tape-recorded during the communicative sessions of mother and child: the babbling and vocalisations increased both in variety and length. Simmons (1964) has described how the first "words" appear, e.g., "meme" for milk, "bah" for bath, etc.

We *conclude*: However slow it may be, in essence it is the same process as the development of the eupraxia of speech in a normally hearing child.

c. The order of difficulty of phonemes in learning to speak

That the eupraxia of speech in deaf children has many similarities with the eupraxia of speech in normally hearing children, also follows from the study of Hudgins and Numbers (1942) about the intelligibility of speech of deaf children. They found an *order of difficulty of phonemes:* some phonemes are easily learned, others not. Typically enough this order is correlated with the frequency of the same phonemes in colloquial language: a rank-correlation of .41 (G. Miller, 1960): the more pronounceable a phoneme is (for deaf children), the more it is used in daily conversations (by the hearing).

d. "Phonetic symbolism", also called "oral mime" (van Ginniken, 1922)

Heider (1940) showed that 32 prelingually deaf adolescents of 16 to 18 years of age could understand the *"phonetic symbolism"* of words, almost in the same way as normally hearing people. At that time hearing aids were not used yet for profoundly deaf children. We confirmed Heider's finding by our investigations (van Uden, 1963).

e. The influence of the hearing aid
The listening behaviour by means of a *hearing aid* is an enormous support to both babbling and lipreading. It has the special advantage of the auditory loop. These effects have been proved by many studies, using tape-recordings, e.g. Ewing (1951), Pickless (1957), Taylor (1960), Downs (1968), Neppert (1969), see also Löwe (1976), Lach et al. (1970), etc.

Summary and conclusion
There is some babbling in congenitally profoundly deaf children, to some extent comparable with the babbling of normally hearing children. It operates like a circle process by means of an articulatory loop. It can be influenced by a constant of the speech from outside, by means of lip-reading and sound perception. There are some similarities between the development and the functioning of eupraxia of speech in prelingually profoundly deaf children and that in normally hearing children.

III. Difficulties in the development of the eupraxia of speech in congenitally profoundly deaf children

We have seen so far that this development is dependent upon these factors:
  the programming of the motor brain;
  the auditory, articulatory and visual control;
  the motor-sensory integration of this whole into one Gestalt.

1. DIFFICULTIES FROM ADDITIONAL HANDICAPS

See the introductory chapter, and chapter I. 3.

2. DIFFICULTIES ORIGINATING FROM THE ATTITUDES OF THE EDUCATORS

Redgate et al. (1972) investigated 245 prelingually deaf children in a longitudinal way for 4 years from 4;6-8 years of age, distributed among 12 schools for the deaf. They found the following factors, apart from the use of a hearing aid and the intelligence, crucial: the interest of the parents, the ability and continuity of the teachers, the zeal of the child himself. – Defeatism or lack of trust, of confidence and optimism are dangerous attitudes.

Many studies have shown how lack of acceptance in the *parents* endangers the growth of language and speech in the deaf child. We mention Oliver (1965), Neuhaus (1969), Luterman (1970), Markides (1972), Schlesinger and Meadow (1972), Greenstein (1975) and many others.

3. DIFFICULTIES DIRECTLY DUE TO DEAFNESS

They may be summarized by the term "delayed speech automation". We mention four typical factors endangering the deaf child:

- Lack of *tempo* of motor behaviour. This has been found by many researchers, e.g., Morsh (1937), Ewing and Stanton (1943, 1957), Myklebust (1964) etc. This may be due to the reaction time, which is longer after a visual than an auditory stimulus (see Woodward-Schlossberg, 1971). How this is mirrored in the speech of deaf children has been found by Hudgins et al. (1942, 1958).
- Lack of *rhythm*. Rosenstein (1957) found deaf children behind normally hearing seeing and blind children, in discriminating vibratory rhythm patterns. (The deaf reacted in the same way as normally hearing sensorily aphasic children.) See further Sterritt et al. (1966), Rileigh and Odom (1972). Beertema (1980) found congenitally profoundly deaf children behind in diadochokinetic syllables (tatatata, kakakakaka, takatakataka etc.). We ourselves (1969, see below) found deaf preschool children significantly behind normally hearing children in imitating rhythmic patterns. Hudgins et al. (1942) showed how this lack of rhythm is mirrored in the speech of the deaf.
- *Breathing* control. From the studies of Teel et al. (1967, cf. Kumpf, 1964) we know that normally hearing people control their breathing not only consciously but also unconsciously. The unconscious breathing of the deaf seems to be normal (cf. Schorsch, 1929). Difficulties appear, however, as soon as the deaf child tries to use his breathing consciously: blowing, blowing the nose and similar (cf. Walther, 1895). Many researches have shown that severe disturbances of breathing control may appear when the child starts to learn to speak (Gutzman, 1905; Hudgins, 1937; Mitrinowitch, 1937; Woldring, 1956; Speth, 1958; Brankel et al., 1965, and many others): especially too high a breathing technique, lack of coordination between the intercostal and the diaphragmal breathing, asymmetric breathing pressure between left and right, polypnoea and tachypnoea etc. "Deafmute-phonasthenia" may be a consequence, hence a falsetto voice too (cf. Zaliouk, 1960). Indirect consequences are: still more difficulty with the rhythm of words and the rhythmic grouping of words into phrases; the deaf person may become too tired from his speech and try to avoid it, etc.
- Too strong a *conscious* control of speech in the beginning. A normally hearing child will start his speaking even when the cortical organisation of his brain is as yet incomplete: he already speaks with subcortical centres, including the limbic system (cf. Dimond, 1980). This may be the origin of typical emotional-automated speech in normally hearing patients suffering from motor aphasia by brain damage. In

48

some way we may say that speech in a normally hearing baby grows from below to above, from an unconscious "steering" towards a conscious control. Later on, especially when he starts to read and write, he reflects upon his own speech, in order to detect how it is composed and structured. Usually this is not so in a prelingually profoundly deaf child. Most speech therapists start their work in a very conscious way, when the child is already 4 or 5 years of age and rather "mute". The way to automation then grows from above to below. This is not a necessity, however. Several speech therapists and phoneticians (e.g. Reichling, 1949; Rosa de Werd, 1964; Ewing, 1964; Ling, 1976; Calvert and Silverman, 1975 and others) have shown that the natural babbling of a deaf child can be guided towards speech by means of classic conditioning and operant conditioning. The consequences of too late a commencement of speech education have been shown by Handsel and Moron (1969, quoted by Kling-hammer, 1971).

- Lack of *frequency* of speech usage. No skill can develop without sufficient repetition and training. Speech cannot be automated without that. See Markides (1976).

Summary and conclusion
One should not close his eyes to the dangerous barrier, congenital profound deafness raises against an achievement of oral communication, i.e., of lipreading-hearing (sound perception) and of intelligible speech. Deaf children need a very cooperative environment and skilful educators.

IV. A survey of methods in teaching deaf children to talk

This topic will be explained to a larger extent elsewhere ("A sound-perceptive method for deaf children", in press). Literature: Haycock (1933, 1954), Reichling (1949), van Uden (1952), Sr. Rosa de Werd (1964), van Dongen (1957, 1962), Berkhout (1968), Kloster-Jensen and Jussen (1970), Clarke School (1970), Calvert and Silverman (1975), Ling (1976), and others.

1. BACKGROUND PRINCIPLES

Speech is not the same as articulation (Reichling, 1949). Articulation is a performance within the breathing muscles, the vocal cords, mouth and nose. Speech is a performance towards others who hear and see the speaker, "a broadcasting" of sounds into an acoustic space. Therefore awareness of sound, both auditory and vibratory, by means of hearing aids, is essential. "Directed towards others" means that the conversational aspect of speech is essential too. A speech therapist, teaching speech merely as articulation, is doing a very bad job and will not have much success, unless the other educators fill in the gap.

2. SPEECH IS A RHYTHMIC BEHAVIOUR "PAR EXCELLENCE" (VAN UDEN, 1952)

It is not possible to develop good speech without a total rhythmic training, both by "sound-perception" and movement. Rhythmic speech is essential for the automation of speech, its intelligibility, its pleasure and harmony, its short- and long-term memory, and last but not least for the structure of language (phrase-structure, "compound construction",

51

"pincer construction", van Uden, 1977). A speech therapist, showing himself satisfied with an articulation as "yes-ter-day" instead of "ye*ss*-terday" is doing a bad job and essentially breaks down the oral attitude of his pupil.

3. A CONTINUAL PROCESS FROM EARLY CHILDHOOD (EWING, 1964)

Muteness can and must be prevented, by guiding the spontaneous babbling, laughing etc. into "vocables" (= incomplete words, Malisch, 1919; Reichling, 1949) and correct words and phrases, by means of classic and operant conditioning.

4. SURVEY OF THE METHODS

a. A method is called *analytic*, if it mainly aims at the articulatory positions, and sees a word as a catenation of those positions (Rogers, 1867; Vatter, 1892; Yale, 1938). The phonemes are mainly taught as kinemes (see above). The self-control, the child primarily learns, is articulatory. Very often, the teacher has to put the articulatory organs into the right positions. Therefore this kind of methods can be called "moulding methods" or "prefabricating methods" ("prefab-methods"). The child is asked to imitate the teacher, more than the reverse. This way of working cannot be applied to very young children, only on the average from about 5 years of age. Reading and writing, connected with this way of speech teaching, is also in the main taught in a graphic-analytic way: words are catenations of letters, each letter or group of letters representing a kineme.

b. The *synthetic* methods see speech primarily as a kind of expressive movement, carrying a meaning, as a "motor-Gestalt". "Vocables" are accepted as incipient words (e.g., bah for ball, cf. Malisch, 1919). Usually the graphic representation of words starts in a "global" way, e.g. ball, to be identified with several objects and pictures. The graphic analysis comes afterwards.

We can distinguish two subdivisions of these methods:

(1) From the outset *the child has to imitate* the teacher (Malisch, 1919; Haycock, 1933; Numbers, 1942, and many others). The teacher may start by using those words which the child already understands through lipreading-hearing and/or has spontaneously imitated.

(2) Particularly, from the outset, *the teacher* does not so much ask the child to imitate him, but most of all *imitates the child*. For example, when conversing with the child about "boots" on a rainy day, and

the child imitates "boa(ts)", he will not try to change "boa" into "boo", but imitates the child: "Yes, boats!" and finds a picture of a boat, giving a meaning to the vocable uttered by the child, forgetting "boots" for a while. He starts conversing with the child about boats on the water, a boat made from paper etc. Perhaps at the moment the child gives a vowel similar to that of ball, the teacher will immediately imitate him, by saying: "Yes, this is a ball!" and will put it into the water, where it will float like a boat. He will try to maintain the difference between "boa(t)" and "ba(ll)". Etc. He follows the course of operant conditioning and classic conditioning (see above). (Reichling-Rosa de Werd, 1949, 1964; Krijnen, 1967, 1972).

Such synthetic methods can also be called: "reactive methods", because they start from and mainly employ the spontaneous reactions of the children, the second sub-division more so than the first one, very suited to children of 1-2 years of age.

The main means of self-control, developed within the child, is the visual and sound perceptive perception by means of amplification, and not so much the articulatory perceptions. This last means of self-control is not neglected but developed afterwards by a mode of *reflecting*, e.g.: "Do you feel the difference between the /K/ in key and in cook?", i.e. how the first /K/ is further to the front of the mouth and the second one more at the back. For this the child has to be at least 5 or 6 years of age.

5. DIFFERENT DEGREES OF TRANSITIVITY

We are able now to compare the different features of speech and the various ways of monitoring it. Speech gives:
an auditory impression, a visual one, a vibratory one, a tactile-kinesthetic one and a very typical tactile one by the use of the Kern-method.

NB. There is another avenue of self-control, however, that of *the tactile sense in the palm of the hand*. This is used in the so-called "Tad-Oma"-method (K. and S. Alcorn 1938, 1941) and still better by Kern's method (1958). The Alcorns make the child feel the teacher's cheek and his own with the palm of his hand, the vibrations of the vocal cords with the little finger and the movement of the lips with the thumb (as is done for deaf-blind children, the first ones having been Tad and Oma). Kern (1958) makes the child speak into the palm of his own hand, developing Barczi's method (1936), also Bieri (1947), Müller and Hägi (1950).The teacher also speaks into the hand of the child, and makes the child compare the teacher's speech and his own alternately, by feeling. It has been found experimentally that all (German) words can be distinguished by the Kern-method. Although Kern himself prefers a synthetic approach, his method can also be used in an analytic way.

All of these impressions are proprio-ceptions and proprio-per-ceptions within our own body. The physiology and psychology of perception rightly distinguishes between so-called "subjective senses" and "objective senses" (cf. Lersch, 1954; Lindsay and Norman, 1973). The latter ones, being the senses of seeing and hearing, affect the perceiving organism much less subjectively than the first, being the senses of touch, including vibration feeling, taste and smell. The more subjectively a movement affects the organism, the more that movement can be called transitive. So washing oneself is a more transitive movement than solo dancing, singing is a more transitive movement than subvocal speaking (lest the articulatory impressions are kept unconscious). Applied to the control of speech: when we articulate in a more pronounced and precise way in a room with a noise that would prevent us from hearing ourselves, *that* speech is more transitive than our normal, mainly auditorily monitored speech, which we would use in a quiet room.

The methods of teaching deaf children to talk, described above, can be arranged according to the degree of the transitivity of speech:

- most transitive seems to be the analytic approach with strong articulatory impressions;
- rather less transitive seems to be the Kern-method;
- still less transitive seems to be the use of visual impressions, e.g. by means of a mirror and/or video-monitoring;
- the least transitive seems to be the method using lipreading and sound perception as the main source of speech control.

Our prime advice to our speech teachers is the following rule:

The more difficulties a deaf child has in his motor control, the more the method of teaching him to talk must include transitive aspects of the speech movement.

The reason is: transitive movements are monitored more easily than intransitive movements.

So a deaf child suffering from a mild dyspraxia will have a need for more use of the mirror and/or video-recording, in order to observe his own speech more throughoutly. (This in addition to a strong training of sound perception and rhythm feeling, which is necessary for all prelingually profoundly deaf children.) A child with a moderate dyspraxia will have a need for more and more elements of the Kern-method, according to the degree of his "speech clumsiness", in addition to the stronger use of visual and auditory feedback. A deaf child suffering from apraxia of speech will have a need for still stronger subjective and transitive impressions of speech: elements of the analytic method, perhaps the analytic method in its entirety, in addition to the stronger visual and auditory feedback and the Kern-method.

6. A DIAGRAM OF THE DIFFERENT METHODS

The speech teachers of the Institute for the Deaf at Sint-Michielsgestel follow an "eclectic" way of teaching, choosing the best out of every method: the methods used are adapted to suit the motor ability of the child.

Figure 7.

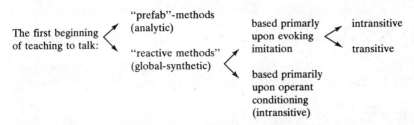

Steps of the "reactive method":
1-2 yrs of age:
1. An oral environment must be established, challenging oral behaviour, first of all developing face-directedness and sound-awareness in the child.
2. "Seizing method" = the parent or caretaker imitates the child as in a babbling game, evoking varieties of babblings, by applying the principle of maximum against minimum contrast (e.g. by presenting suddenly "bowow" after "mama"), gradually decreasing the contrasts.
3. He makes the child enjoy the *auditory* function by means of the hearing-aid (many deaf children can learn to respond to their names) and the auditory feedback, e.g. by making the child manipulate sounding toys, and enjoy *visual* feedback by making the child use a mirror and manipulate a lamp in his mouth, etc.
4. He makes the child enjoy long babblings (e.g. yayayayaya), and trains the breathing and the rhythm.

1¹/₂-3 yrs of age:
5. Meaningfulness: the parent or caretaker attaches meanings
   • to babblings, by means of which they may grow to "vocables" (as "bowow"),
   • to words, word groups, so-called "accent groups", as ballballball, ballcarball, carcarball etc. (cf. nursery rhymes) because of the rhythm and the breathing,

55

- to sentences as "Hello Peter!" "Want marmelade!" "Thank you! "Going to play" "I'am going to play" etc.
- to oral-aural conversations.
6. He applies classic and operant conditioning.

2½-4 yrs of age:
7. He introduces speech-balloons as "deposits" for the memory (speech is not meant to be taught from the written forms here): he writes down
   - vocables as BRRR (cold!), MMM (delicious!), OOH! (how big!), Bowow, hello!
   - words and sentences, which are eventually written as "visualized conversations".
8. He develops differentiations and sequences of speech, integration of the spoken and the written forms, auditory discrimination, etc.

7. THE GRAPHIC SUPPORT

Normally hearing people very often need a graphic support for the building up of an exact image of a word or expression. When we hear a new word, unknow to us, e.g. "eclecticism", we very often ask: "How do you write it?" The written form is a help not only to our memory but also to our correct pronunciation, especially for the right order of the phonemes.

Exactly the same happens with deaf children: the greater their hearing loss, the more a graphic support is necessary. In our opinion this has to start at the earliest stages, i.e. in the preschool years by parents' guidance, which in our program is referred to as "hometraining": parents are instructed to keep diaries (cf. Dale, 1968). This reading can begin at about 2½ years of age (van Uden, 1978) in a very informal and playful way. For example, a child of 2½ years of age was looking at a fish in his father's aquarium and then said to his mother: "Papa!" (Daddy), meaning: "That fish is saying papa". The fish was opening and closing its mouth, and to the child this was indeed "papa". Immediately the mother drew it for him in the diary (Figure 8):

The speech-balloons are very helpful. The child understands: what is written there, is the same as what is spoken. This can grow towards small "visualized conversations", such as shown in Figure 9.

A typical phenomenon appears now:
For some children, those who experience difficulty in lipreading, this written form can become a stepping stone towards lipreading. Rather

56

Figure 8.

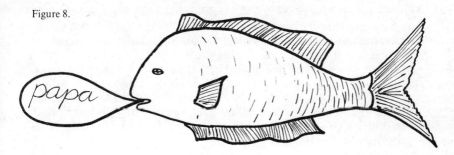

Figure 9.

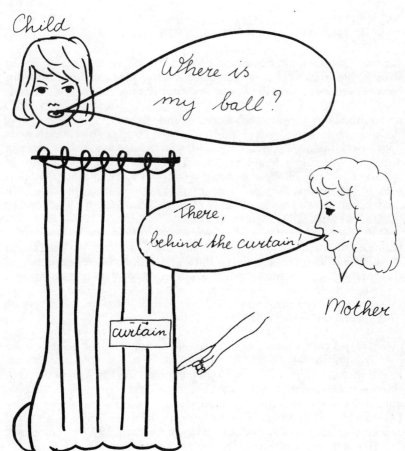

57

often one sees that very quickly these children become interested in the written form. This seems to be due to the "syndrome of dyspraxia" (usually inclusive of a strong memory for *simultaneously* presented data), which is the main topic of this study.

At about 4 1/2 years of age a kind of "draw-writing", ususally spontaneously, starts, i.e. a writing which is closely connected with drawing.

At 5 1/2-6 years of age the "reading vocabulary" (data Institute for the Deaf Sint Michielsgestel, the Netherlands, van Uden, 1974) comprises about 600-1000 words, the "writing vocabulary" (i.e. writing from memory) about 60-100 words.

8. SOME DATA ABOUT THE *SPEECH* OF CONGENITALLY PROFOUNDLY DEAF CHILDREN IN THE INSTITUTE FOR THE DEAF AT SINT-MICHIELSGESTEL

We will discuss: spontaneous non-conversational vocalisation, tempo of speech, oral technical communicative ability, short-term memory for spoken sentences, oral digit span and oral fluency.

a. Spontaneous vocalisation: deafness and silence?
Prelingually profoundly deaf children between the ages of 4 and 18 years with a performance IQ greater than 80 who indulge, on the one hand: in vocal plays, whistling, humming, and on the other hand: in production of unconscious oral sounds and speaking without voice to other deaf persons, have been investigated by means of an inquiry among the care staff, qualified in the education of the deaf at the residence of the school for the deaf at Sint-Michielsgestel (1972).

Only those children have been involved who could be educated orally, without esoteric means of fingerspelling and/or signing. We have divided them into two groups, with a third group as a control-group:
(A) prelingually profoundly deaf children, 4-18 years of age, without speech difficulties: 134;
(B) prelingually profoundly deaf children, 4-18 years of age, with speech difficulties: 87;
(C) severely hard of hearing children (60-90 dB loss, Fletcher index, ISO), 12-18 years of age: 57 (multiply handicapped ones, coming from other schools).

For the statistical comparisons we computed the Chi square distribution (χ^2) on the raw scores. For a better readable comparison we converted the raw scores into percentages.
(1) "Does this child *vocalize for his own pleasure* using vowels and consonants, outside the conversational situation?" Percentages of the number of children who do are shown in Table 10.

Table 10.

Ages	4;6 – 6;5	6;6 – 8;5	8;6 – 10;5	10;6 – 12;5	12;6 – 14;5	14;6 – 16;5	>16;6	χ^2
A. Deaf children without speech difficulties	88.2	52.6	64.3	57.7	41.4	36.8	20.0	22.34 df. 6 $p<0.01$ S.
B. Deaf children with speech difficulties	77.8	76.2	33.3	50.0	18.1	33.3	9.1	25.8 df. 6 $p<0.01$ S.
C. Severely hard of hearing children	–	–	–	–	66.7	60.0	16.0	12.7 df. 2 $p<0.01$ S.

ΣA and ΣB χ^2 3.05 df. 1 p = 0.09 Tendency.
3 ages $\Sigma A+B$ and ΣC χ^2 11.127 df. 1 p < 0.01 S.

The numbers of children using vocal play appear to be significantly related to the age, for all groups: the numbers decreased according to the age. Many deaf toddlers vocalize in the evening in bed, before going to sleep and while sleeping in dreams.

There appears to be no significant difference between A and B, but a significant difference of the three ages A + B with C, i.e. from 12;6 through > 16;6 years of age.

(2) "Does this child *whistle* for his own pleasure?" Percentage of the number of children who do are given in Table 11.

There appears to be no significant difference between the groups A and B, but there are significantly more hard of hearing children whistling than deaf ones.

(3) "Does this child *hum* for pleasure?" Percentages of the number of children who do are shown in Table 12.

There appears to be no significant difference between A and B.
There appears to be a significant difference between the two groups of deaf children and the group of severely hard of hearing children.

(4) "Does this child make oral sounds *un*consciously?" Percentages of the number of children who *often* do are to be found in Table 13.

59

Table 11.

Ages	4;6 – 6;5	6;6 – 8;5	8;6 – 10;5	10;6 – 12;5	12;6 – 14;5	14;6 – 16;5	≥16;6	χ^2
A. Deaf children without speech difficulties	0.0	5.3	7.1	30.8	37.9	21.0	30.0	14.043 df. 6 p<0.05 S.
B. Deaf children with speech difficulties	0.0	28.6	33.3	25.0	27.3	22.2	27.3	2.383 df. 6 p = 0.89 N.S.
C. Severely hard of hearing children	—	—	—	—	44.4	53.3	36.0	1.664 df. 2 p = 0.44 N.S.

ΣA and ΣB χ^2 0.708 df. 1 p = 0.41 N.S.
3 ages ΣA+B and ΣC χ^2 3.948 df. 1 p < 0.05 S.

Table 12.

Ages	4;6 – 6;5	6;6 – 8;5	8;6 – 10;5	10;6 – 12;5	12;6 – 14;5	14;6 – 16;5	≥16;6	χ^2
A. Deaf children without speech difficulties	11.8	10.5	42.9	50.0	20.7	15.8	20.0	15.85 df. 6 p < 0.01 S.
B. Deaf children with speech difficulties	22.2	23.8	15.1	50.0	18.1	22.2	18.2	6.496 df. 6 p = 0.37 N.S.
C. Severely hard of hearing children	—	—	—	—	55.6	66.7	36.0	4.129 df. 2 p = 0.13 N.S.

ΣA and ΣB χ^2 0.363 df. 1 p = 0.55 N.S.
3 ages ΣA+B and ΣC χ^2 20.499 df. 1 p < 0.01 S.

There appears to be a tendency of difference between the deaf children and the hard of hearing ones, the numbers of the latter being smaller.

There does not appear to be a significant difference between the groups A and B.

Table 13.

Ages	4;6 – 6;5	6;6 – 8;5	8;6 – 10;5	10;6 – 12;5	12;6 – 14;5	14;6 – 16;5	⩾16;6	χ^2
A. Deaf children without speech difficulties	17.6	5.3	28.6	19.2	20.7	5.3	30.0	6.961 df. 6 p = 0.33 N.S.
B. Deaf children with speech difficulties	11.1	19.0	22.2	25.0	45.5	33.3	18.2	5.748 df. 6 p = 0.46 N.S.
C. Severely hard of hearing children	—	—	—	—	11.1	13.3	12.0	0.014 df. 2 p = 0.99 N.S.

ΣA and ΣB χ^2 0.854 df. 1 p = 0.36 N.S.
3 ages ΣA+B and ΣC χ^2 3.674 p = 0.06 Tendency

(5) "Does this child talk *voicelessly* to *other* hearing impaired persons?"
Percentages of the number of children who *often* do are given in
Table 14.

Table 14.

Ages	4;6 – 6;5	6;6 – 8;5	8;6 – 10;5	10;6 – 12;5	12;6 – 15;4	14;6 – 16;5	⩾16;6	χ^2
A. Deaf children without speech difficulties	23.5	21.0	35.7	50.0	20.7	21.0	40.0	7.404 df. 6 p = 0.29 N.S.
B. Deaf children with speech difficulties	22.2	23.8	33.3	25.0	45.5	33.3	18.2	3.529 df. 6 p = 0.74 N.S.
C. Severely hard of hearing children	—	—	—	—	22.2	13.3	16.0	0.703 df. 2 p = 0.70 N.S.

ΣA and ΣB χ^2 0.445 df. 1 p = 0.51 N.S.
3 ages ΣA+B and ΣC χ^2 3.026 p = 0.08 Tendency

There appear to be no significant differences between the groups A and B. There is a tendency, however, that less hard of hearing than deaf children speak voicelessly to other hearing impaired persons.

b. Tempo of speech

Van Balen (1974) investigated the tempo of speech from radio-recordings, calculating the speed, ignoring the pauses. He found an average tempo, which he calls a normal tempo, of 6.4 syllables per second ±1.3. Where the tempo exceeded 7.8 syllables, it was considered very quick; if it did not reach 5.0 syllables, it was considered very slow. But the tempo as such did not influence the intelligibility. The same has been found by Pickett and Pickett (1963).

We measured the tempo of speech from television broadcastings, and tape-recorded class-room conversations of teachers and prelingually profoundly deaf children, at the ages 9, 11 and 12 years. We found three kinds of varieties of rate, see Table 15.

Table 15.

Syllables and pauses	Very quick tempo, usually that of "news readers"	moderate tempo, as in quiet conversations	"solemn" tempo, as that of "declaimers" of poetry and of preachers
Average number of syllables per second, ignoring the pauses	7.15 ± 0.76	5.23 ± 1.55	2.60 ± 3.23
Average number of syllables, pauses of speech included	4.29 ± 0.84	3.14 ± 2.10	1.56 ± 2.78

The "solemn" tempo appeared to be more variable, according to moods and feelings.

The tempo of the deaf children was as shown in Table 16.

In general we may say that the deaf children in this investigation spoke in a "solemn tempo", comparable to that used by preachers and public speakers. The rate of utterance is slower than that used by normally hearing people in conversation.

Table 16.

Syllables and pauses	Deaf children of 9 years of age	Deaf children of 11-12 years of age
Average number of syllables per second, ignoring the pauses	2.54 ± 2.00	3.07 ± 2.56
Average number of syllables per second, speech pauses included	1.44 ± 2.38	2.30 ± 3.21

c. Short-term memory for speech

This is part of the routine-testing of our deaf children. Apart from the "lipreading-hearing-imitating test", two further tests are used: one for the short-term memory of spoken sentences, and the "digit-span"-subtest of the Wechsler Intelligence Scale for Children (1949).

The "18 syllable sentence test", which originated in Sint Michielsgestel, has been translated into English for this book. It must be standardized if the Englisch version is to be applied. The reliability has been calculated from the scores of 24 prelingually profoundly deaf children of different ages, by a comparison of two experimenters, the author and Miss Georgette Claes, psychological associate. The "split half"-correlations were .91 and .87 respectively. The test-retest reliability was .84 and .86 respectively. The experimenter U. van C.-correlation was test .72, and retest .78 respectively. All of these correlations were significant (p < 0.001).

Facing the child, the experimenter has to utter the sentences in a clear "solemn" and rhythmical manner, from memory. The head should be kept still, and normal facial expression used. He closes his eyes, in order to make the child concentrate fully on his speech. Lighting should be normal, so that shadows are avoided. The child wears his individual hearing aid, and sits at about 1.50 meters from the experimenter. He is not allowed to read the sentences, and the experimenter must be very careful to ensure that the child will not see the typed sentences and read them upside down.

NB. Prelingually profoundly deaf children can be educated in such a way that they memorize words mainly by an articulatory coding (Conrad, 1970, 1979; Thomassen, 1970). For a critical summary of these studies see van Uden (1977).

64

Figure 10.

Test containing ten 18-syllable non-compound sentences. – Each time, the experimenter says the sentence once, maintaining the marked intervals. He writes down what the child repeats. The correct syllables are counted, irrespective of the sequence.

Number of correct syllables:

1. On Wednesday morning / we will be going / to and from Southampton / by bus. ——— ———
2. In the tall trees / hundreds of birds were playing / on this beautiful morning. ——— ———
3. Whose turn is it today / to take the dinner down / to the two sick children? ——— ———
4. The train to London / will be leaving / at a quarter past nine / to-morrow. ——— ———
5. Mummy wanted to buy / ten oranges at seven pence each / from the shop. ——— ———
6. I like nice weather / during the holiday, / lots of sunshine and no rain. ——— ———
7. Mummy, / is Mary allowed / to put so much sugar / on her sandwiches? ——— ———
8. Grandmama and Grandpapa / have a big kennel / and seven puppy-dogs. ——— ———
9. The cat / has been sitting under the tree / all evening / to catch a mouse. ——— ———
10. Why / are the seven airplanes on the airfield / making such terrific noise? ——— ———

Average number of correct syllables:

"Digit span": the way of testing is the same as with the 18 syllable sentences, but according to the instructions and scorings of the WISC, see Chapter VI.

Figure 11.

●——●: correctly repeated syllables from 18 syllable sentences.
O——O: correctly repeated series of digits, forward and backward (rough scores), according to the Wechsler Intelligence-Test for Children (WISC).

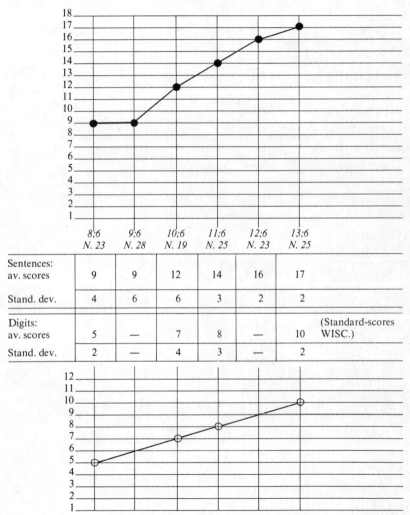

	8;6 N. 23	9;6 N. 28	10;6 N. 19	11;6 N. 25	12;6 N. 23	13;6 N. 25	
Sentences: av. scores	9	9	12	14	16	17	
Stand. dev.	4	6	6	3	2	2	
Digits: av. scores	5	—	7	8	—	10	(Standard-scores WISC.)
Stand. dev.	2	—	4	3	—	2	

d. Oral technical communicative ability and oral fluency

Figure 12.

"Lipreading-hearing-imitating-test": see p. 104-105.

Lipreading test with sound perception and repeating.

N.B. The words need not be known to the children.

Words	Score:	Loose speech sounds:	Repetition from memory					Correct speech sounds:
			1	2	3	4	5	
1. whip (1)(3)	0-1-2-3-4							1
2. pat (1)(3)	0-1-2-3-4							2
3. bell (1)(3)	0-1-2-3-4							3
4. big (1)(3)	0-1-2-3-4							4
5. young (1)(3)	0-1-2-3-4							5
6. stood (1)(4)	0-1-2-3-4							6
7. table (2)(5)	0-1-2-3-4							7
8. tam-tam (2)(6)	0-1-2-3-4							8
9. comma (2)(4)	0-1-2-3-4							9
10. tearing (2)(5)	0-1-2-3-4							10
11. cold (1)(4)	0-1-2-3-4							11
12. mason (2)(5)	0-1-2-3-4							12
13. apple-sauce (3)(7)	0-1-2-3-4							13
14. assistant (3)(8)	0-1-2-3-4							14
15. lavatory (4)(8)	0-1-2-3-4							15
16. deliverance (4)(10)	0-1-2-3-4							16
17. dance (1)(4)	0-1-2-3-4							17
18. stand (1)(5)	0-1-2-3-4							18
19. grand (1)(5)	0-1-2-3-4							19
20. grip (1)(4)	0-1-2-3-4							20
21. kilogram (3)(8)	0-1-2-3-4							21
22. independency (5)(12)	0-1-2-3-4							22
23. automatic (4)(8)	0-1-2-3-4							23
24. extra (2)(6)	0-1-2-3-4							24
25. hotel (2)(5)	0-1-2-3-4							25

Words	Score:	Loose speech sounds:	Repetition from memory					Correct speech sounds:
			1	2	3	4	5	
26. plastic (2) (7)	0-1-2-3-4							26
27. commandant (3) (9)	0-1-2-3-4							27
28. tendency (3) (8)	0-1-2-3-4							28
29. tomato (3) (6)	0-1-2-3-4							29
30. stock-still (2) (8)	0-1-2-3-4							30
31. stable (2) (6)	0-1-2-3-4							31
32. quartz (1) (6)	0-1-2-3-4							32
33. left (1) (4)	0-1-2-3-4							33
34. glad (1) (4)	0-1-2-3-4							34
35. tremendous (3) (9)	0-1-2-3-4							35
36. propaganda (4) (10)	0-1-2-3-4							36
37. historian (4) (9)	0-1-2-3-4							37
38. electric (3) (8)	0-1-2-3-4							38
39. openmindedness (5) (13)	0-1-2-3-4							39
40. supplement (3) (9)	0-1-2-3-4							40
41. comprehensible (5) (14)	0-1-2-3-4							41
42. handiness (3) (8)	0-1-2-3-4							42
43. horizontal (4) (10)	0-1-2-3-4							43
44. aviary (4) (6)	0-1-2-3-4							44
45. dishonesty (4) (9)	0-1-2-3-4							45
46. immoderate (4) (8)	0-1-2-3-4							46
47. candelabra (4) (10)	0-1-2-3-4							47
48. abstract (2) (8)	0-1-2-3-4							48
49. anatomical (5) (10)	0-1-2-3-4							49
50. hullabaloo (4) (8)	0-1-2-3-4							50

TOTAL

TOTAL SCORES: _____ — total of loose speech-sounds: _____ = _____

_____% of the 200.

68

Figure 13.

● = Lipreading with sound perception and repeating.
o = Speaking as many words as possible within 2 minutes.

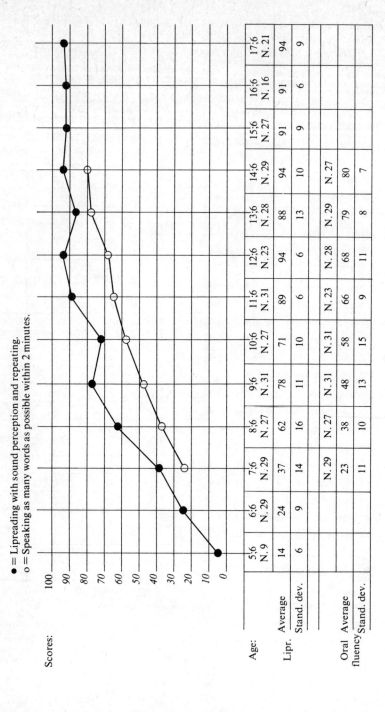

Age:		5;6 N. 9	6;6 N. 29	7;6 N. 29	8;6 N. 27	9;6 N. 31	10;6 N. 27	11;6 N. 31	12;6 N. 23	13;6 N. 28	14;6 N. 29	15;6 N. 27	16;6 N. 16	17;6 N. 21
Lipr.	Average	14	24	37	62	78	71	89	94	88	94	91	91	94
	Stand. dev.	6	9	14	16	11	10	6	6	13	10	9	6	9
Oral fluency				N. 29	N. 27	N. 31	N. 31	N. 23	N. 28	N. 29	N. 27			
	Average			23	38	48	58	66	68	79	80			
	Stand. dev.			11	10	13	15	9	11	8	7			

Scores: 100 90 80 70 60 50 40 30 20 10 0

The three tests mentioned above have been used in our research on the syndrome of dyspraxia. Digit span, oral fluency, lipreading-hearing-imitating-test and the last part of this test "repetition from memory" have been put together and their function has been called:
"Supple use of the mouth when speaking"
Ages of the children: 7 through 10 years, 1973. See Chapter VI. Cf. Lancioni (1981).

The sum-scores of test (5) "repeating spoken series of digits", (13) "saying as many words as possible within 2 minutes", (14) "Lipreading-hearing-imitating", and (15) "repetition of correctly imitated words", which give an indication of the child's ability in "supple use of the mouth when speaking", were compared with the daily "oral behaviour" at home and in the school residence. The extent to which speech and possibly miming, gesturing and signing were used, was investigated by means of three questionnaires, the answers to which could be scored, with a maximum score of 12 each, total sum 36 max.

The results were as follows:

(1) Oral behaviour and environment
There were three kinds of environments as far as communication was concerned (Table 17):
    deaf parents ($N = 5$);
    hearing parents with more than one deaf child ($N = 23$);
    entirely hearing environment ($N = 55$).

Table 17.

Groups	Oral behaviour at home max. 12	Oral behaviour in residence	
		with supervisors max. 12	among themselves max. 12
Deaf children from deaf parents	9.53	9.83	8.00
Deaf children with deaf brother or sister	9.12	9.62	8.14
No other deaf person in family	9.42	9.27	8.29

There appeared to be no difference between the groups as regards oral behaviour. There was, however, a tendency ($p < 0.09$) that the children

69

communicated less orally with each other than with the parents (inclusive of deaf parents) and with the supervisors in the residence.

(2) Comparison of the sum-scores of the five tests mentioned with the three inquiries on oral behaviour

We have to take into account below that the tests were taken on average 2-3 years earlier than the inquiries. The correlations per group (9 groups) were as follows: (0.46) – (0.21) – (0.53) – (0.24) – (0.63) – (0.47) – (0.49) – (0.26) – (0.37).

These correlations per group were not significant, because the groups were too small. All the groups together ($N = 83$) gave 0.43 $p < 0.01$.

Summary and conclusion

There seems to be no reason for pessimism or defeatism in the teaching of speech to deaf children. The difficulties mentioned above can be overcome. This conquest seems to be dependent more upon the skill, the art of the teachers than on the ability of their children, although the latter plays an important part. This will be the topic of the next chapters: the syndrome of dyspraxia.

V. Disturbed psychomotor development and congenital deafness. An introductory study (1971)*

1. CONGENITAL DEAFNESS AND EURHYTHMIA

We applied a test for eurhythmia (1955) to three groups of children, 3;6 to 6;5 years of age, by tapping on a table and saying "baba" in different rhythmic patterns. The results (maximum score 40) are shown in Table 18.

Table 18.

A. Congenitally deaf, n = 36:	27.71 ± 8.11
B. Hearing losses between 75 and 85 dB (including children with progressive deafness), n = 14:	32.66 ± 4.21
C. Children with normal hearing, n = 11:	39.66 ± 0.51

A < B t = 2.1244 p < 0.05
B < C t = 2.7175 p < 0.02

We thus found a significant backwardness in deaf children with respect to eurhythmia. This is in agreement with daily experience. This backwardness can be corrected, however, in a cybernetic way. In a pilot study done on two groups of deaf children, we found (1955, 1963) that melodies played on "blow-organs" with electronic amplification by the children themselves (group I) were recognized better than the same melodies played to them by another person (group II). Moreover, the first group showed spontaneous rhythmic movements of the trunk and the arms during the recognition task, but the second group did not.

* Published in G. B. A. Stoelinga and J. J. van der Werff ten Bosch (eds.) "Normal and abnormal development of brain and behaviour", Martinus Nijhoff Publishers B.V., The Hague 1971, p. 250-256, reproduced here (with a few adaptations) by the courtesy of both editors and publishers.

2. EUPRAXIA AND EURHYTHMIA AND CONGENITALLY DEAF CHILDREN

We constructed a test for eupraxia (1970). This test measures the speed in location of arms and legs and fingers, for intransitive movements. We found a significant and high correlation between this eupraxia and eurhythmia as measured by these tests. Both are correlated to speech-reading and to memory for spoken sentences (1968), as shown in Table 19.

Table 19. Matrix of correlations. Prelingually deaf children, n = 60, aged 10,0 - 17,11 years.

	Eurhythmia	Speech-reading	Memory for sentences	Mental age
Eupraxia	0.85 (p < 1%)	0.76 (p < 1%)	0.62 (p < 1%)	0.14 (N.S.)
Eurhytmia	——	0.77 (p < 1%)	0.67 (p < 1%)	0.20 (N.S.)
Speech-reading		——	0.77 (p < 1%)	0.31 (p < 2%)
Memory for sentences			——	0.49 (p < 1%)

3. DYSPRAXIA, DYSRHYTHMIA AND "MOTOR-DYSPHASIA"

On the basis of these findings, we were able to predict difficulties for deaf children in learning to lipread, to talk and to benefit from auditory training.

When deaf children are found to score below the 25th percentile rank of the tests for eupraxia and eurhythmia, within the population of deaf children of the mental ages 3;6-5;6, typical difficulties in speech can be expected (with related difficulties in speech-reading and auditory training):

a. perseverations of phonemes, e.g. lomonade;
b. inversions of phonemes, e.g. melonade;
c. cut-offs, e.g. lemade;
d. difficulties in short-term memory, i.e. a continuous deterioration in the production of words and phrases when the child is requested to repeat them from memory e.g. (5 times) lemonade, lomade, lomo, lamo, lo...

We measured this last finding by counting the total omissions of phonemes within these five repetitions (Table 20).

Table 20.

Loss of phonemes in a speech memory test		
Deaf children < 25 th perc. rank	83% ± 19	
Deaf children > 25 th perc. rank	27% ± 21	t = 6.2500 p<1%

This disturbance is a kind of dyspraxia of speech, or "motor-dysphasia" (Prick and van der Waals, 1958, 1965; Luchsinger and Arnold, 1970). All this can also happen in children with high intelligence.

Methods of teaching to talk should be adapted to such children. On the basis of our findings, programmes for training in eurhythmia (1968-1969, Erlangen 1971), control of the body scheme, serial successive memory, and integration of movements with graphic symbols have been developed or are in various stages of development in our Institute.

The number of deaf children (in our Institute) who show this multiple handicap of deafness and "motor-dysphasia" amounts to 20-25% of the prelingually deaf (data 1971), who are mostly successfully educated in a purely oral way. Only in exceptional cases the disturbance is so severe that alternative means of communication, e.g. speech and fingerspelling, sometimes even fingerspelling only, should be included.

4. A TYPICAL PROFILE OF LEARNING APTITUDE IN DEAF CHILDREN WITH DYSPRAXIA, INCLUDING DYSRHYTHMIA

The Nebraska non-verbal test of learning aptitude (1966) was applied to two groups of 16 deaf children aged 4;6-9;6, one composed of dyspraxics and the other of eupraxics. These groups were matched according to age, deafness, and non-verbal intelligence (Performance IQ) (Table 21).

Table 21.

	Eupraxics (n = 16)	Dyspraxics (n = 16)	t	Significance
Chronological age	7.11 ± 1.6	7.2 ± 2.4	0.0300	NS
Performance IQ	103 ± 8.74	107 ± 11	1.0282	NS
Learning age	7.6 ± 2.4	7.8 ± 1.8	0.1170	NS
Eupraxia	101 ± 13.41	48 ± 18.26	9.0750	p < 1%
Eurhythmia	117 ± 41.78	40 ± 16.69	6.7662	p < 1%
Speech-reading	49.18 ± 21.14	15.17 ± 13.32	6.320	p < 1%

The Hiskey-Nebraska test (1966) for these ages comprises eight sub-tests.
1. Imitation and memory of Bead Patterns.
2. Memory for Colours.
3. Picture Identification.
4. Picture Association: the child is requested to find the correct picture according to some relation, e.g. Figure 14.
   The child has to fill in the picture of a flying kite.

Figure 14.

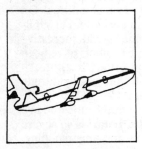 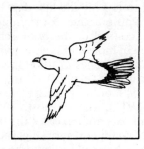 

5. Paper Folding: the child has to remember and imitate a series of paperfolding movements.
6. Visual Attention Span: the child has to remember series of pictures presented simultaneously.
7. Block-Patterns.
8. Completion of Drawings.

For each subtest, the raw scores are converted into an "age", in months. The median age of these 8 "ages" is the "learning Age". The other "ages" are scattered around this "Learning Age". We calculated the means of the "ages" of the subtests of both groups separately based on a comparison of an assumed mean of 96 months, to permit comparison which would illustrate the difference between the two groups. The results are plotted in two bar diagrams (see Figure 15), the length of the bars indicating the deviation from the median age ("Learning Age").

Profile of the learning aptitude according to the Hiskey-Nebraska Test (1966). The lengths of the bars indicate the deviation from the average "Learning Age".

The difference between the two groups is significant in:

subtest 5 "Paper folding"
subtest 4 "Picture association"⎫
 The eupraxics score significantly higher than the dyspraxics.

Figure 15.

Profile of the learning aptitude according to the Hiskey-Nebraska Test (1966).
The lengths of the bars indicate the deviation from the average "Learning Age".

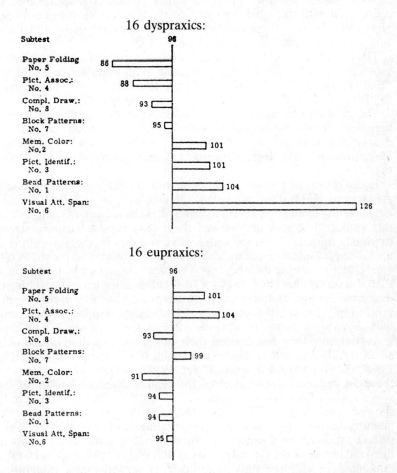

16 dyspraxics:

Subtest	
Paper Folding No. 5	86
Pict. Assoc.: No. 4	88
Compl. Draw.: No. 8	93
Block Patterns: No. 7	95
Mem. Color: No.2	101
Pict. Identif.: No. 3	101
Bead Patterns: No. 1	104
Visual Att. Span: No. 6	126

16 eupraxics:

Subtest	
Paper Folding No. 5	101
Pict. Assoc.: No. 4	104
Compl. Draw.: No. 8	93
Block Patterns: No. 7	99
Mem. Color: No. 2	91
Pict. Identif.: No. 3	94
Bead Patterns: No. 1	94
Visual Att. Span: No.6	95

subtest 1 "Bead patterns"
subtest 6 "Visual attention span"

The eupraxics score
significantly lower than the
dyspraxics.

The unusually high score of the Visual Attention Span (subtest 6) is very
striking. These dyspraxic deaf children generally have a very good
memory for simultaneously presented unrelated visual data. On the one

75

hand this offers a guideline for their educational treatment: by means of "graphic conversation", i.e. using their strong side as a compensatory factor. On the other hand these children seem to be "absorbed" into a kind of "visual-image-thinking", a direct "visualizing behaviour". In connection with this, their insight into the invisible relations between pictures (subtest 4) is underdeveloped, and they have many difficulties with successive memory (subtest 5) too.

The profile of the dyspraxic deaf children is significant with respect to: subtest "Attention Span" (6) in contrast to all other subtests; subtest "Bead Patterns" (1) and subtest "Picture Identification" (3) in contrast to "Paper Folding" (5) and "Picture Association" (4).

The profile of the eupraxic deaf children is only significantly prominent for: "Picture Association" (4) – one of the weak sides of the dyspraxic deaf children – in contrast to "Memory Color" (2), "Picture Identification" (3), "Bead Patterns" (1), and "Visual Attention Span" (6).

In the course of 8 years 89 children with *normal pure-tone threshold audiograms* and normal nonverbal intelligences, aged 3;4-10;7 years, but suffering from some learning disabilities, have been investigated by this author. The vast majority of them (54) suffered from a strong dyspraxia-apraxia combined with a weak auditory memory, resulting in a weak speech-memory, as measured by the Digit-span test of the WISC and (Dutch) sentence memory test. Their speech-memory correspond to that of severely deaf children (with 70-90 dB hearing losses), resulting in dysgrammaticism, as appearing in an utterance like this: "Bump he, my arm bump!" These children show a lack of ability to speak grammatically. The reason seems to be obvious: after two or three words they have forgotten how they had started their utterance and therefore cannot structure it in a correct sentence (van Uden, 1977). These children suffer from "developmental dysphasia" (cf. Wyke, 1978). The majority of these 54 children clearly showed the typical cognitive profile of the syndrome of dyspraxia described above. Of the other 35 children 17 showed some degree of dyspraxia but none the less a normal speech-memory because of a strong, compensating auditory memory. They suffered more from a sensori-motor integration disturbance. Most of them did not show the typical profile of the syndrome of dyspraxia. (The remaining 18 children only suffered from sensori-motor integration problems.) (Table 22).

NB. The *profile* of a strong "Picture Identification" in contrast to a weak "Picture Association" has not been confirmed by my further investigations. Therefore it has not been incorporated in the next research, described in chapter VI. It seemingly has to do with another disorder: a sensori-motor integration disturbance with as consequence integrative dyslexia and dyssymbolia, see above (cf. van Uden, 1980).

76

Table 22.

Children	With the cognitive profile of the syndrome of dyspraxia	Without the cognitive profile of the syndrome of dyspraxia	Total Numbers
Children with a weak speech-memory	42	12	54
Children with a normal speech-memory	4	13	17
Total numbers	46	25	71

χ^2 16.684 df. 1 p < 0.01
The distribution appears to be significant.

Analogous data are found in Stevens (1975), Both (1982) and Van Dijk (1982).

Summary and conclusion
Auditory disorders seem to be connected with specific disturbances in motor and cognitive behaviour. This calls for special programs of basic training in eurhythmia, eupraxia, serial successive memory, integration of motor behaviour (including speech) and of movement associated with symbols (including verbalisations).

There is, however, no reason for pessimism in view of the results shown by many well-educated deaf children.

On the contrary, improved diagnosis of these problems in deaf children may lead to an improvement in the educational treatment of them.

VI. The "syndrome of dyspraxia" in some prelingually profoundly deaf children. – Can tests given to deaf children shed any light on their difficulties in learning to speak?

Introduction

One of the tasks of the deaf children's psychologist is to discover the factors which influence speech-training either favourably or unfavourably. For this purpose a great number of tests are given to the children, 15 of which are, as indicated by experience, especially concerned with speechtraining, apart from residual hearing and intelligence.

At the ages of between 6 and 11, deaf children's speech develops quickly. In these years they proceed from "ideovisual" to "receptive" reading, resulting in the first reading-book for hearing children being dealt with in the class at the age of about 9 to 10, which development has a particular influence on the content of speech and the extension of the vocabulary (Sint Michielsgestel, data by IJsseldijk, see van Uden, 1977).

1. QUESTION

The question posed is as follows:

How do the results of these 15 tests interrelate and how do they relate in connection with speech of non-multiply handicapped deaf children aged between 6 and 11 years?

2. SUBJECTS

There were 147 children available, all of the Institute for the Deaf, Sint Michielsgestel (schoolyears 1966-1972). From these 83 were chosen as complying with the following criteria: they had to be aged between 7 and 10 years; they had to be strictly prelingually profoundly deaf and have a performance IQ of 90 or more, with hearing-loss and intelligence distributed homogeneously; they had to have had hometraining from the latest age of 3 and to have attended the "changing class" of the Institute, i.e. with one week's admission into the observation department, at least twice before their 4th birthday; they had to have finished in the nursery school for deaf children within 2 or 3 years and to have been admitted to the primary school for the normal deaf; no children who had multiple defects which would have necessitated admission into a special class were included in the study; they had to have been for at least 2 years reasonably or well educated – according to circumstances – by an experienced teacher; they had to have had an oral education without supplemental sign language or fingerspelling; – we had to be sure that at home too they lived in an oral environment.

The *etiology* of their deafness, according to the medical histories, was as shown in Table 23.

Table 23.

Etiology	Eupraxia	Slight dyspraxia
Meningitis in the first year of life	4	3
Maternal rubella	1	4
Anoxia at birth?	0	1
Heredity	24	17
Born deaf, cause unknown	11	18

One looked for a connection, if any, between this etiology and eupraxia or dyspraxia. No such connection was found.

The division of boys and girls was as follows (Table 24).

Table 24.

		Eupraxia	Slight dyspraxia
Girls		21	16
Boys		21	25
	Total	42	41

Some discrepancies in the selection of subjects have to be mentioned. In each age-group there was one child with a slight form of integration-dyslexia, i.e. a difficulty of integration of the spoken and the written form of words. – In the group of 8 year olds, there were two children with a multiple handicap, which was not too severe, however.

Thus we were able to form four age-groups which did not differ significantly as regards hearing-loss and performance-intelligence, see Table 25.

Table 25.

Group	Age	Number of children	Boys	Girls	Prelingual hearing-loss in dB	Wechsler performance IQ	Hiskey derived IQ
I	7;0- 7;11	20	12	8	100.1±11.3	106.4± 9.4	108.5±14.9
II	8;0- 8;11	18	8	10	108.8±10.5	106.3±12.5	108.4±10.7
III	9;0- 9;11	23	14	9	108.9±10.5	107.0±10.6	104.0±12.3
IV	10;0-10;11	22	12	10	110.0± 9.3	108.7±12.8	104.3±12.3
I-IV	7;0-10;11	83	46	37	108.5±10.3	107.1±11.2	106.1±12.6

3. THE 15 TESTS

(1) Remembering simultaneously presented coloured rods (Hiskey's test, 1966 "memory for colours"). Abbreviated to *Si.C.*
The experimenter holds two sets of eight coloured rods. He puts one set in front of the child. After the child has had a good look at the rods, the experimenter covers them with cardboard. Then he shows one rod from his own set for 2 seconds, after which he takes the cardboard away to cover this one rod. At the same time the set of eight rods which are lying in front of the child becomes visible again. The child now has to select the rod having the same colour as the one which was shown to him from the experimenter's set, and put it aside. After that the experimenter takes the cardboard away from the rod which he showed. The child can now see whether his choice was right or wrong. This is repeated eight times with one rod, three times with two, twice with three rods etc. up to and including twice with six rods. The selections must always be completely correct. The score per time is 1 or 0. Maximum score: 19.

(2) Imitating demonstrated successive folding movements (Hiskey's test, 1966 "Paper folding"). Abbreviated to *Su.Fo.*

The experimenter picks up a sheet of paper and folds this in a certain way. Then he gives a similar sheet to the child, who has then to imitate the same folding movements from memory. At first this is done twice with one folding movement, then twice with two movements, and then each time once with from three up to and including seven movements. The score per time is 1 or 0. Maximum score: 9.

(3) Remembering simultaneously presented pictures (Hiskey's test, 1966 "visual attention span"). Abbreviated to *Si.Pi.*

The same procedure as described under (1) is followed, this time using pictures. The number of pictures from which the child has to choose is gradually increased, from 6 to 12 to 18. Again the experimenter begins with one picture, then two etc. up to and including seven. The score is 0 when one picture is wrong, 1 when all the pictures have been remembered but not the correct order, and 2 when the order is correct too. Maximum score: 16.

(4) Remembering successively presented pictures. Abbreviated to *Su.Pi.*

Immediately after test (3) the experimenter repeats this same test, but shows the pictures from the series 2 up to and including 7 successively, each picture for one second. Each series is shown twice in succession so that each picture is seen for two seconds. The scoring is the same as for (3).

(5) Repeating spoken series of digits (Wechsler's test WISC, 1949 "Digit span" Dutch standardisation). Abbreviated to *Di.Sp.*

The experimenter speaks a series of numbers first, without the child being able to see the written images. The length of the series varies from 3 up to and including 9. After that a second series follows with 2 up to and including 8 numbers, the child having to repeat the series in reverse order. The score is either 1 or 0. Maximum: 17.

(6) Simultaneous digit/symbol association (Wechsler's test WISC, 1966 "coding") Abbreviated to *D.sy.*

NB. Since we are not allowed to reproduce the test itself here, we have chosen symbols different to the ones used in the WISC coding-test.

The child receives the following model (Figure 16), which he keeps in front of him during the whole of the test:

Figure 16.

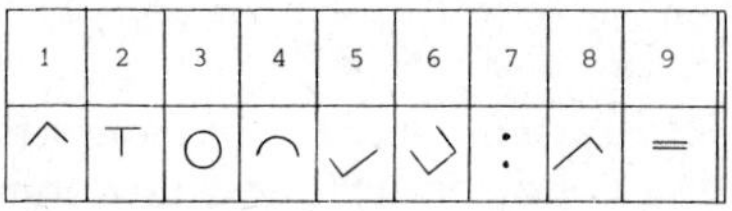

1	2	3	4	5	6	7	8	9	
∧	T	○	⌒	✓	↺	:	∧	=	

For exercise-purposes he receives the following model, Figure 17:

Figure 17.

2	3	1	5	4	9	6	8	7	3	1	etc.

Following this the test starts with Figure 18.

Figure 18.

Within 2 minutes the child has to fill in correctly as many consecutive symbols as possible. Maximum: 57.

(7) Copying simultaneously presented geometrical figures from memory (Benton's test, first presentation 1953). Abbreviated to *Bt.C.*
The experimenter shows the child a geometrical figure on a card for 10 seconds. After that he takes the card away, gives the child a sheet of paper of the same size and asks him to copy the figure from memory. There are 10 such cards. The first two show only one figure, the other 8 show three. The score is either 1 or 0. Maximum: 10.

(8) Identifying simultaneously presented geometrical figures from memory (Benton's test, second presentation 1953). Abbreviated to *Bt.Id.*
Immediately after test (7) is finished, (8) is presented. The same cards are again shown for 10 seconds. This time, however, the child does not have to copy them, but is shown another card, on which there are four similar figures, of which only one is the same as that on the card shown. He has to indicate the identical figure. The scoring is the same, i.e. either 1 or 0. Maximum: 10.

(9) Tapping successively four cubes in a shown order (Knox's Cube test, 1914, standardisation in Snijders-Oomen, 1970). Abbreviated to *Knox*.

The child has, from left to right, 4 cubes in front of him, 5 centimeters apart. The experimenter, with another cube, taps some of them successively, e.g. 1-3-4, in a tempo of 1 tap per second. After that he gives his cube to the child, who has to copy these movements. There are 15 series, first of 2 taps, then of 3 etc. up to and including 6. The score is either 1 or 0. Maximum score 15.

(10) Putting the fingers in a certain position according to an example (Bergès and Lézine's test, 1963 "Imitation of gestures"). Abbreviated to *Bergès*.

The experimenter puts his fingers in a certain position and keeps them like that, until the child has imitated him. We refined the original scoring as follows. One hand is not allowed to help the other. If the child cannot imitate the position of the fingers without some help, the score is 0. If the child does not put his fingers in the correct position within 5 seconds, but puts it right finger by finger, the score is $1/2$. If the child manages to get it right within 5 seconds, the score is 1. Maximum score: 16.

The standardisation on deaf children is shown in Table 26, Figure 20.

Test of finger-eupraxia for intransitive movements

Name of Child: ....

Date of Test: ....

Age: ....

Name of Examiner: ....

A. Adapted test of Bergès and Lézine (1963, Paris): 2nd part = positions of fingers.

Drawings by the courtesy of Mason Co. Paris.
Photo VandeWal.

1. The investigator shows a particular position of his hand(s). This must be done in such a way that the child does not see *how* he does it. The investigator has to know the position by heart, so that he is able to show it *quickly*. If the investigator has some difficulty himself, he has to "construct" the position outside the view of the child, f.i. under the table.

2. The investigator requests the child to imitate the hand position; not by heart = the investigator keeps his position until the child has imitated it, unless it becomes clear that the child is unable to do it. There is no time limit.
3. The child is allowed to use his right or left hand; but if he has imitated the investigator's right hand with his left hand (mirror position), he has to use the other hand for the left hand of the investigator. (Until ± 9 years of age, the child is expected to use mirror positions, never beyond that age. If it does, and/or if it is not consistent in its right-left use, this is a sign of trouble within the control of the body scheme.)
4. Instruct the child that it *is not allowed* to *help* its one hand with the other; each hand has to find its own position.

Scoring: If the child achieves the positioning *immediately,* i.e. at least within 5 seconds, it scores *1 point.*
If it has to try to correct and/or "*construct*" its finger-positions, but finally succeeds, it scores $^1/_2$ *point.*

Figure 19.

Items:		5	
2-2	$0 - \frac{1}{2} - 1$	1 ◇	$0 - \frac{1}{2} - 1$
1-1	$0 - \frac{1}{2} - 1$	∞	$0 - \frac{1}{2} - 1$
$\frac{2}{1}$ ◇	$0 - \frac{1}{2} - 1$	▽	$0 - \frac{1}{2} - 1$
L. V	$0 - \frac{1}{2} - 1$	X	$0 - \frac{1}{2} - 1$
R. V	$0 - \frac{1}{2} - 1$	⊏⊐	$0 - \frac{1}{2} - 1$
L. ♂	$0 - \frac{1}{2} - 1$	⊏⊐	$0 - \frac{1}{2} - 1$
R. ♂	$0 - \frac{1}{2} - 1$	8	$0 - \frac{1}{2} - 1$
L. ⊔	$0 - \frac{1}{2} - 1$	Score:_____	
R. ⊔	$0 - \frac{1}{2} - 1$	(max. 16)	

See p. 86-90.

Table 26.
Standardization of Bergès and Lézine's test of handpositions, (van Uden, 1967):

Age	Number of children involved	Average score
3 yrs.	5	3 ± 1
4 yrs.	21	7 ± 1
5 yrs.	18	9 ± 2
6 yrs.	23	11 ± 4
7 yrs.	27	12 ± 3
Ceiling: 8 yrs.	27	14 ± 3
9 yrs.	30	14 ± 3
10 yrs.	22	16 ± 3

NB. Deleau (1978) did not find any difference between deaf and normally hearing children on this test.

Figure 19 continued.

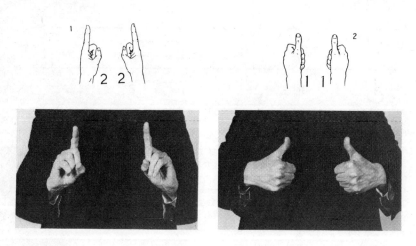

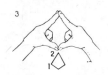

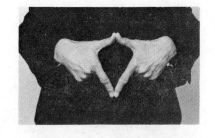
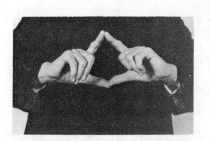

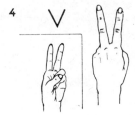
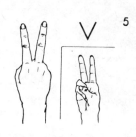

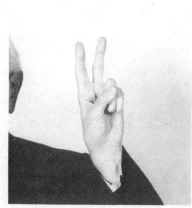
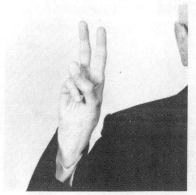

87

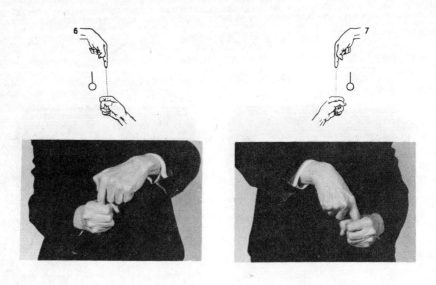

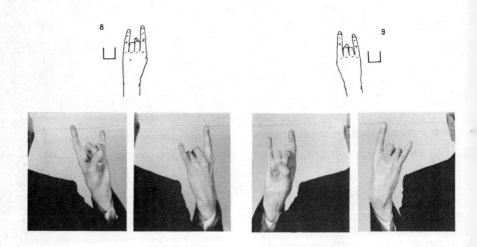

88

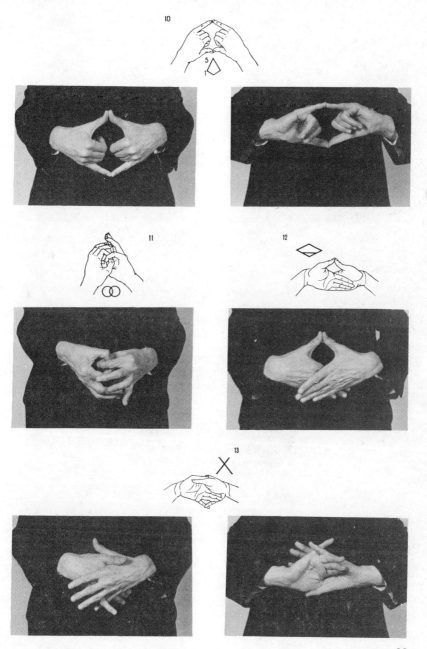

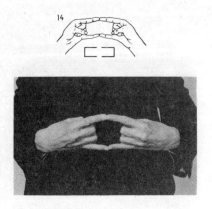

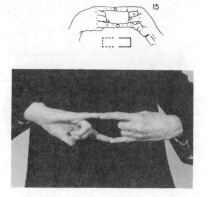

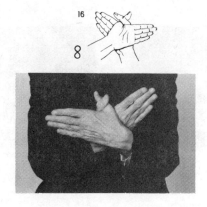

Figure 20

Standardisation of Bergès and Lézine's test of handpositions.

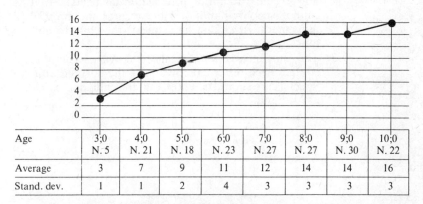

Age	3;0 N. 5	4;0 N. 21	5;0 N. 18	6;0 N. 23	7;0 N. 27	8;0 N. 27	9;0 N. 30	10;0 N. 22
Average	3	7	9	11	12	14	14	16
Stand. dev.	1	1	2	4	3	3	3	3

(11) Imitating shown finger-movements from memory (Van Uden's test, 1967), Abbreviated to *Fi.Mov.*

The experimenter puts his hand or hands up, behind his head, so that he cannot see his own fingers. He then touches the tip of his thumb with the tip of his index-finger three times. The child is asked to imitate this without looking at his fingers. Next the experimenter does the same with the middle-finger, then with the ring-finger and the little-finger; then all fingers in a row, at first in a tempo of 1 second per touch, then of $1/2$ a second, then of $1/4$ a second. The score is 0 if the child uses the wrong finger(s), 1 when he touches the right finger but not the finger-tip, 2 if both aspects are correct. Maximum score 42. See p. 92-96.
Standardization on deaf children in Table 27, Figure 22.

(12) Repeating rhythmically spoken syllables (Van Uden's test 1970, second part.) Abbreviated to *Rhythm.* See p. 100-102.

The experimenter first says the following rhythmic pattern: ba-babá. He closes his eyes, in order to attract the full attention of the child to his speaking lips. The child has to repeat this pattern. The score is 0 if the pattern is unrecognisable, 1 if it is recognisable but when the metre is not quite correct, 2 if everything has been repeated correctly. This is repeated once again. After this the child is asked to repeat the pattern five times without help. Each time the scoring is worked out in the same way. The rhythmic patterns increase in difficulty, for example baba-bababá, babababá etc. There are 15 items. Maximum score 210. Standardization on deaf children in Table 29. Continue on p. 104.

B. Imitating Finger movements from memory (Van Uden, 1967)

Instruction: 1. The investigator puts the hand or hands in question upward, next to and a little *behind* his head so that he cannot see his hand(s). He executes the prescribed movement. *After* that he requests the child to imitate him.
2. The movements involve the *fingertips*. These must contact each other exactly and in the correct tempo.
3. Special care should be taken that the child does *not look* at his hand.

Figure 21.a

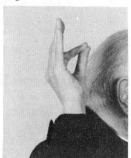

Scoring: Perfect imitation *2 points*. The right finger(s) move(s), but the contact of the fingertips is not quite exact, and/or more fingers move together to the opposite thumb, and/or the child corrects himself spontaneously and similar, *1 point*. – The child does not use the right finger(s), *0 point*.

N.B. For the items 5-13: Sometimes the child does not stretch the fingers after a movement, but pushes the 4 fingers over the thumb. The investigator must correct it. If the child continues doing so, it is *0 point*. Sometimes the child bows its finger(s) too much, without moving it (them) towards the thumb. The score can be 2 points, but we note it down, because it can be an indication of lack of differentiation (*immaturity*) of motor control. This is just a clinical note. – For the items 1-4 and 11-13: the movements left and right should be synchronic = *eutaxic*. The score can be 2 points, but we note it down, just as a clinical observation of dystaxia.

I. Fingertip of *one* finger with the thumb tip (both hands synchronically)
1. 3 times the *forefinger-tip* contacts the *thumb-tip*; before and after this the hand is *stretched* (see photographs):

92

$$0 - 1 - 2 \quad 0 - 1 - 2 \quad 0 - 1 - 2 \quad = \ldots \ldots \text{points (max. 6)}$$
2. The same with the *middle-finger:*
$$0 - 1 - 2 \quad 0 - 1 - 2 - \quad 0 - 1 - 2 \quad = \ldots \ldots \text{points (max. 6)}$$
3. The same with the *ring-finger:*
$$0 - 1 - 2 \quad 0 - 1 - 2 \quad 0 - 1 - 2 \quad = \ldots \ldots \text{points (max. 6)}$$
4. The same with the *little-finger:*
$$0 - 1 - 2 \quad 0 - 1 - 2 \quad 0 - 1 - 2 \quad = \ldots \ldots \text{points (max. 6)}$$

II. Successively – forefinger, middle-finger, ring-finger, little-finger; before and after each movement the hand is *stretched* (see photographs):

5.	R.	*Tempo*	1	second	per finger –			0 – 1 – 2
6.	L.	,,	1	,,	,,	,,		0 – 1 – 2
7.	R.	,,	1/2	,,	,,	,,		0 – 1 – 2
8.	L.	,,	1/2	,,	,,	,,		0 – 1 – 2
9.	R.	,,	1/4	,,	,,	,,		0 – 1 – 2
10.	L.	,,	1/4	,,	,,	,,		0 – 1 – 2
11.	R.+L.	,,	1	,,	,,	,,		0 – 1 – 2
12.	R.+L.	,,	1/2	,,	,,	,,		0 – 1 – 2
13.	R.+L.	,,	1/4	,,	,,	,,		0 – 1 – 2

$$\Sigma \ldots \ldots$$
$$\text{(max. 42)}$$

Total Score:
Bergès   . . . .
Van Uden . . . .
Σ . . . .
(max. 58)

Table 27.
Standardization of van Uden's fingermovements test (van Uden, 1967).

Age	Number of Children Involved	Average Score
7 yrs.	27	27 ± 9
8 yrs.	31	31 ± 9
9 yrs.	20	33 ± 7
10 yrs.	22	34 ± 6
Ceiling:		
11 yrs.	20	38 ± 6

94

Item 1 - 13 fingertip of *one* finger with the thumb-tip, behind the head, so that the hand cannot be seen; before and after this the hand is stretched.

Figure 21b.

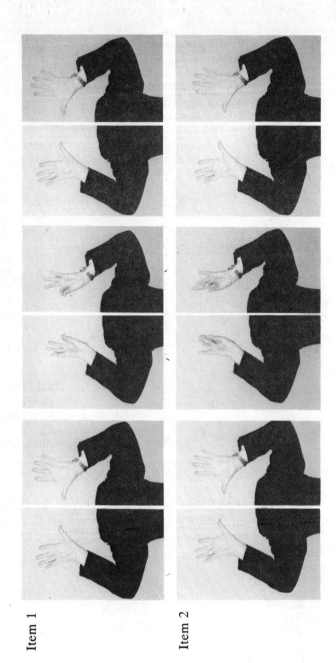

Item 1

Item 2

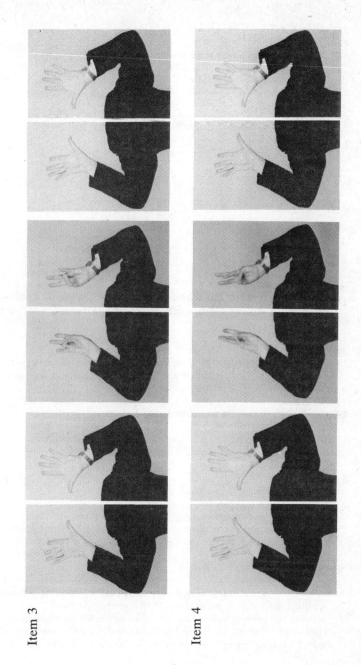

Item 3

Item 4

Figure 22

Standardisation of van Uden's fingermovements test (1967)

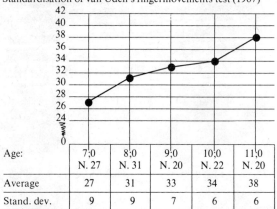

Age:	7;0 N. 27	8;0 N. 31	9;0 N. 20	10;0 N. 22	11;0 N. 20
Average	27	31	33	34	38
Stand. dev.	9	9	7	6	6

A. A rhythm test for hand and mouth for prelingually profoundly deaf preschool children 3;6 - 6;5 years of age (van Uden, 1969).

Name of child   : . . . .
Date of test   : . . . .
Age: . . . .   Name of examiner: . . . .

Scores: 0 = no or unidentifiable reaction, different from the model.
        1 = rather good, acceptable reaction, tempo included.
        2 = an excellent raction.

NB. Examiner and child sit at a table facing each other.   *Score:*

1. The examiner says, with eyes closed, with a tempo of one second:
   ba...ba...ba...ba...ba...etc. about 7-8 times. The child is invited to imitate
   him, with eyes closed.   0 – 1 – 2

2. Idem, with a tempo of ¹/₄ second.   0 – 1 – 2

3. The examiner gives the child a *peg*. He himself has a peg too. He taps
   with the peg on the table, upon one point, without saying ba ba, tempo of
   1 second. The child is invited to imitate him.   0 – 1 – 2

4. Idem, with a tempo of ¹/₄ second.   0 – 1 – 2

---

5. a. With the *peg:* the examiner taps on one point of the table, twice ●●, with a tempo of
   ¹/₄ second. Immediately after tapping the pattern he puts his hand upwards, so that the
   rhythmic unit appears well-bound. The child now holds his peg in his preferred hand
   (right or left). The examiner holds that hand and demonstrates the rhythmic pattern by
   tapping ●● upon one point of the table. Straight away, he raises the child's hand.

96

Then, or at the same time, he shows the pattern himself again with his own hand (= the preferred hand of the child). Then the child is invited to imitate him independently. Maximum of 5 trials. After one success (score 1 or 2) he shows the child how to do it 5 times in repetition. He invites the child to do the same, that is to repeat the pattern from memory 5 times.

    a. Pattern ●● (¹/₄ second)   0–1–2 1...2...3...4...5...= score... (max. 10)
    b. Idem: ● ● (1 second)   0–1–2 1...2...3...4 ..5,,.= score... (max. 10)
    c. Idem: ●●● (¹/₄ second) 0–1–2 1...2...3...4...5...= score... (max. 10)

6. Idem, but now the patterns are tapped in a *spatial* way, that is not tapping on one point but on different points of the table, ●● close to each other at a distance of about 2 inches, and ● ● at a distance of about 10 inches.

    a. Pattern ●● (¹/₄ second)   0–1–2 1...2...3...4...5...= score... (max. 10)
    b. Idem: ● ● (1 second)   0–1–2 1...2...3...4...5...= score... (max. 10)
    c. Idem: ●●● (¹/₄ second) 0–1–2 1...2...3...4...5...= score... (max. 10)

7. Now the same patterns with *baba*. The examiner takes away the pegs. He shows the pattern with his eyes closed, opening them after the pattern has been accomplished, so that the child is aware of the rhythmic unit. Maximum of 5 trials. After one success (score 1 or 2) he shows how to do it 5 times: he closes his eyes and says baba, waits about 2 seconds, repeats it, etc., opening his eyes after the fifth repetition.

    a. Pattern: baba (¹/₄ second) 0–1–2 1...2...3...4...5...= score... (max. 10)
    b. Idem: ba..ba (1 second)   0–1–2 1...2...3...4...5...= score... (max. 10)
    c. Idem: bababa (¹/₄ second) 0–1–2 1...2...3...4...5...= score... (max. 10)

Total (max. 26):...Total repetitions (max. 90)...

___

8. *Integration* with a graphic symbol. The examiner takes 3 blanc cards of 2 by 10 inches. He draws a circle O (symbolising ●●) in the middle of the card, saying baba, showing the symbol next to his mouth, saying again baba. He puts this card on the table to his left side. – Then he takes the second card and draws a square □ (symbolising ●.....●), saying ba.....ba, showing the symbol next to his mouth, and puts this card in front of him. Then the same with bababa and a triangle △ (symbolising ●●●), putting that card on the right side. Figures 23 and 24.

Figure 23

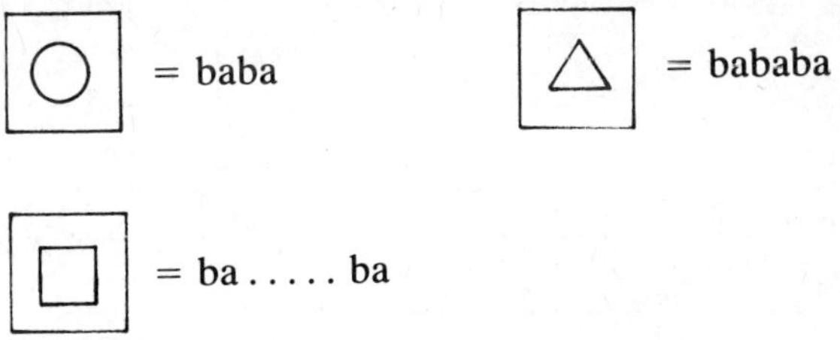

    O = baba   △ = bababa

    □ = ba . . . . . ba

Figure 24

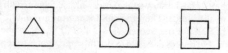

Then he shows the cards again in turn next to his mouth, inviting the child to imitate him. After this he puts the cards on the table in a random order and then says baba. He invites the child to say baba and mimes the question saying: "Show me the card!". The child has to point to the correct card. If the child fails, he is corrected and is shown the correct card. Then the experimenter takes away the cards, puts them again on the table in a different order and says ba...ba, acting in the same way. After that the same follows for bababa. – Finally he examines the child, without giving any corrections, taking away the cards, putting them on the table again and again in an other order. The items are:

Figure 25

baba   ba . .ba   bababa   ba . .ba   baba   bababa   bababa

Score:
0 – 4 – 5 – 6 – 7 (scores 1, 2, 3 are zero because p > 1%).

9. *Integration* continued. The examiner puts the cards on the table in this order:

Figure 26

He points to the first card, inviting the child to say something without showing the model. If the child says baba it is reinforced, if not the mistake is corrected. He does the same with the other two cards. After that he invites the child to point to a card, asking the examiner to say something, thus turning the roles. Finally he examines the child, taking away the cards and putting them on the table again and again in a different order. The items are:

Figure 27

baba   ba . .ba   bababa   ba . .ba   baba   bababa   bababa

98

Score:

0 – 4 – 5 – 6 – 7 (scores 1, 2, 3 are zero because p > 1%)

Σ score integration: ..... (max. 14).

Total (max. 40):.......
Total number of repetitions (max. 90):.......

N.B. The repetitions of part 5, 6 and 7, and the integration subtest part 8 and 9 have not been standardized yet. They can be used only in an experimental and clinical way, in an analogy to part 11 and to the "Lipreading-hearing-imitating-test".

Standardisation of the rhythm test for prelingually profoundly deaf *preschool* children of normal intelligence who have had adequate auditory training (max. score 26):

Table 28.

Age	Number of children involved	Average score
3 years	20	20 ± 4
4 years	27	22 ± 3
5 years	26	23 ± 3
ceiling: 6 years	28	25 ± 3

Figure 28

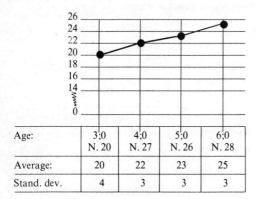

Age:	3;0 N. 20	4;0 N. 27	5;0 N. 26	6;0 N. 28
Average:	20	22	23	25
Stand. dev.	4	3	3	3

B. A rhythm test for oral movements for prelingually profoundly deaf children of 6-12 years of age.

10. *Repeating rhythmically spoken syllables*
This test is executed by asking the child to repeat the syllables "baba" in different rhythmic patterns. The test is stopped when the child cannot do this with three consecutive items at the first and second presentation.

Score
0 = no or entirely wrong reaction;
1 = a reasonably good reaction; the elements are grouped, but the tempo-division is not quite correct;
2 = an entirely correct reaction.

a. One should hide the graphic symbols from the child. Each pattern is only spoken once for one scoring.
b. After the first reaction the child's memory is tested: the rhythm pattern is again spoken and repeated and after this the child is asked to repeat this pattern 5 times from memory. Each time one scores 0 or 1 or 2.

Rhythm pattern:	Score	2nd time	Memory Repeating from memory:
1. ba babá • •é	0 - 1 - 2	0 - 1 - 2	1...2...3...4...5... = score ... (max. 10).
2. babá ba ba •é • •	0 - 1 - 2	0 - 1 - 2	1...2...3...4...5... = score ... (max. 10).
3. babá ba babá •é • •é	0 - 1 - 2	0 - 1 - 2	1...2...3...4...5... = score ... (max. 10).
4. bababá ba •••é •	0 - 1 - 2	0 - 1 - 2	1...2...3...4...5... = score ... (max. 10).
5. ba bababá • •••é	0 - 1 - 2	0 - 1 - 2	1...2...3...4...5... = score ... (max. 10).
6. bábababá é•••é	0 - 1 - 2	0 - 1 - 2	1...2...3...4...5... = score ... (max. 10).
7. bababá babá •••é •é	0 - 1 - 2	0 - 1 - 2	1...2...3...4...5... = score ... (max. 10).
8. babá bababá ba •é •••é •	0 - 1 - 2	0 - 1 - 2	1...2...3...4...5... = score ... (max. 10).
9. bababá babá ba •••é •é •	0 - 1 - 2	0 - 1 - 2	1...2...3...4...5... = score ... (max. 10).
10. bábabábabá é•é•é	0 - 1 - 2	0 - 1 - 2	1...2...3...4...5... = score ... (max. 10).
11. ba bababábá • ••••é	0 - 1 - 2	0 - 1 - 2	1...2...3...4...5... = score ... (max. 10).
12. bababábá babá ••••é •é	0 - 1 - 2	0 - 1 - 2	1...2...3...4...5... = score ... (max. 10).
13. ba bababábá babá • ••••é •é	0 - 1 - 2	0 - 1 - 2	1...2...3...4...5... = score ... (max. 10).
14. bababá ba babá ba •••é • •é •	0 - 1 - 2	0 - 1 - 2	1...2...3...4...5... = score ... (max. 10).
15. ba babá bababá ba • •é •••é •	0 - 1 - 2	0 - 1 - 2	1...2...3...4...5... = score ... (max. 10).

Total: ....
                max. 30   max. 30   max. 150

The max. score of 26 of the test for deaf infants, aged 3 - 5 is added to this:

Total (max. 210): .....
+ 26
―――――
Sum total (max. 236): .....

Table 29.
Standardisation of the rhythm test for prelingually profoundly deaf children of 6-12 years age, of normal intelligence, who have had adequate auditory training, not severely multi-handicapped:

Age	Number of children involved	First presentation (max. 30)	Second presentation (max. 30)	Repetition from memory (max. 150)	Total score (max. 210)
± 6 yrs	33	10 ± 6	14 ± 5	70 ± 21	94 ± 30
7 yrs	38	12 ± 6	14 ± 4	70 ± 18	96 ± 26
8 yrs	33	14 ± 5	18 ± 4	90 ± 17	122 ± 24
9 yrs	37	22 ± 8	26 ± 6	129 ± 30	177 ± 31
10 yrs	33	23 ± 8	26 ± 4	130 ± 18	179 ± 28
ceiling: 11 yrs	29	25 ± 9	28 ± 7	134 ± 24	187 ± 37
12 yrs	30	28 ± 7	30 ± 6	142 ± 23	200 ± 35

Figure 29

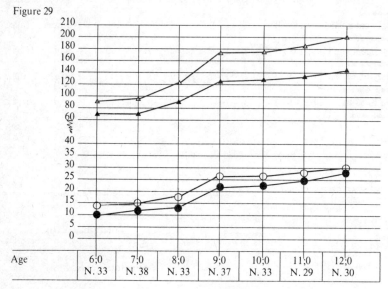

Age

| | 6;0 N. 33 | 7;0 N. 38 | 8;0 N. 33 | 9;0 N. 37 | 10;0 N. 33 | 11;0 N. 29 | 12;0 N. 30 |

● = first presentation   O = second presentation
▲ = repetitions   △ = total score

102

C. *Integration* of a rhythmic oral pattern with a graphic symbol.

Reading.

11. The patterns are symbolised by dots on cards. Subtests nos. 8 and 9 are repeated. Then the cards 1 through 15 are shown to the child, without the examiner speaking them. The child is invited to read the pattern for 3 seconds and to speak it from memory.

	Reading symbol from memory	
Pattern:	After a look for 3 sec.	Repeat by heart
1. • •́	0 - 1 - 2	1...2...3...4...5...= score...(max. 10)
2. •́ • •	0 - 1 - 2	1...2...3...4...5...= score...(max. 10)
3. •́ • •́	0 - 1 - 2	1...2...3...4...5...= score...(max. 10)
4. ••́ •	0 - 1 - 2	1...2...3...4...5...= score...(max. 10)
5. • ••́	0 - 1 - 2	1...2...3...4...5...= score...(max. 10)
6. •••́	0 - 1 - 2	1...2...3...4...5...= score...(max. 10)
7. ••́ •́	0 - 1 - 2	1...2...3...4...5...= score...(max. 10)
8. •́ ••́ •	0 - 1 - 2	1...2...3...4...5...= score...(max. 10)
9. ••́ •́ •	0 - 1 - 2	1...2...3...4...5...= score...(max. 10)
10. ••••́	0 - 1 - 2	1...2...3...4...5...= score...(max. 10)
11. • •••́	0 - 1 - 2	1...2...3...4...5...= score...(max. 10)
12. •••́ •́	0 - 1 - 2	1...2...3...4...5...= score...(max. 10)
13. • ••••́ •́	0 - 1 - 2	1...2...3...4...5...= score...(max. 10)
14. ••́ • •́ •	0 - 1 - 2	1...2...3...4...5...= score...(max. 10)
15. • •́ ••́ •	0 - 1 - 2	1...2...3...4...5...= score...(max. 10)
	..... max. 30	..... max. 150.

12. **Transposing** a spoken rhythm into a graphic symbol. The examiner speaks the rhythms tabulated below by saying baba etc. He folds the paper in order to hide the symbols from the child. The child imitates the examiner, and is then invited to write down the symbols to the right of the line.

Pattern:	Notations of the child:
1. ba ba babá	
• • ••	
2. babá babá ba	
•• •• •	
3. babá ba ba babá	
•• • • ••	

103

4. babá bababá babá

   •• ••• ••

---

5. babababá

   ••••

---

6. babababá bababá

   •••• •••

Score: ... (max. 6).

NB. The subtest C part 11 and 12 have not been standardized yet. It can only be used in an experimental and clinical way at the moment.

(13) Speaking as many words as possible within 2 minutes. Abbreviated to *Or.Fl.* (oral fluency).
The child is asked to speak different words, as many and as quickly as possible. They need not be correctly articulated, provided they are understandable to the experimenter. See above p. 66-68.
Maximum score ± 90.

(14) Lipreading with sound-perception and repeating (van Uden's Test 1970 "Lipreading-hearing-imitating-test" first part). Abbreviated to *Lipr.* See p. 66-68.
The child sits opposite the experimenter at a distance of about $1\frac{1}{2}$ meter. Before the test starts one checks whether the setting of the hearing-aid is correct. The experimenter puts four words in front of the child: *pet – banana – bear – Peter,* words which even the deafest child of these ages is able to distinguish, by sound perception, if the hearing-aid is functioning correctly. He points to the words and asks the child whether his hearing-aid is all right. Then he pronounces these words, one after the other. After that the child has to close his eyes and the experimenter says for example *bear,* after which the child repeats this word and points it out. Next the experimenter asks again if the hearing-aid is all right, i.e. whether it is set as the child wants it. If necessary the three other words are used too in order to achieve the correct setting.
Following this the test proper starts, in which the child continually combines lipreading and sound-perception. The test consists of 50 words, varying from one syllable up to and including five syllables. The scoring is as follows: if the child repeats the word in the correct rhythm after having heard it once, he receives 4 points; if he repeats all the speech-sounds, however, in a less correct rhythm, he is awarded 3 points; if the experimenter only has to say one syllable again and if the

104

child then repeats the whole word correctly, he scores 2 points; should the experimenter have to analyse the word further and the child manages to repeat the word correctly after that, he receives 1 point; in all other cases no points are awarded. Maximum score $200/2 = 100$.

(15) Speaking correctly repeated words again from memory (van Uden's Test 1970 "Lipreading-hearing-imitating-test" second part). Abbreviated to *Spe. rep.*

This is the second phase of test (14): when the child has repeated a word correctly, he is asked to repeat this word up to five times. The experimenter writes down the correct speech-sounds. The score is expressed in percentages of correct speech-sounds.

4. WORKING METHOD

All the tests were individually administered by one and the same experimenter (the author), in a time-span of at most three days per child. The child always wore his hearing-aid.

Ewing (1957) says that anyone who tests deaf children should be fully familiar with these children, because otherwise too many measuring errors arise, e.g. poorly understood instructions, uncertainty in the child, etc. We add to this that the experimenter should be aware of the following peculiarities which can occur in deaf children: they may read the text upside down; they may be strongly influenced emotionally by the scoring; they may, at a glance, notice the direction in which the experimenter is looking (when for example the experimenter involuntarily looks at the picture in question, the child soon sees this and executes the task faultlessly); they may not make a distinction between left and right; they may also slow down their tempo when the experimenter seems disinterested, etc.

We have taken all these into account to the best of our ability when carrying out this experiment.

5. RESULTS

The scores of the 83 children are reproduced in Tables 30-33. We have made up product-moment-correlation matrices per group, as well as of the total. See Tables 34-38.

Table 30

Group I. 7;0 – 7;11, N. 20, 12 boys – 8 girls. "Raw scores".

	1b.	2b.	3b.	4b.	5b.	6b.	7b.	8b.	9b.	10b.	11.b	12b.	13g.	14g.	15g.	16g.	17g.	18g.	19g.	20g.
1. Remembering simultaneously presented coloured rods.	13	14	14	13	13	13	13	15	14	14	13	15	15	13	13	15	14	12	15	16
2. Imitating shown successive folding movements.	7	4	3	6	7	6	7	5	7	6	6	7	4	6	7	7	4	6	8	5
3. Remembering simultaneously presented pictures.	9	9	8	8	8	7	8	10	8	8	8	9	9	7	8	9	9	7	9	11
4. Remembering successively presented pictures.	8	6	5	5	7	5	7	6	8	5	4	8	6	5	6	8	5	6	8	9
5. Repeating spoken series of digits.	5	3	0	5	3	3	5	3	3	0	5	5	3	3	5	6	3	0	6	5
6. Associating simultaneous digit-symbol.	38	21	30	26	29	24	31	37	26	37	30	37	41	23	24	39	41	24	42	45
7. Copying simultaneously presented geometrical figures from memory.	4	5	3	2	3	2	3	4	2	2	3	4	4	2	2	4	3	2	4	7
8. Identifying simultaneously presented geometrical figures from memory.	7	6	6	3	4	4	4	6	5	5	4	5	6	5	5	7	6	4	8	10
9. Tapping four cubes in a shown order.	10	7	6	9	9	9	10	9	8	9	7	10	6	9	10	12	7	7	12	8
10. Putting the fingers in a certain position according to an example.	13	10	11	14	12	13	15	10	10	11	11	12	10	13	14	12	11	12	16	10
11. Imitating shown finger-movements from memory.	31	19	23	38	26	24	38	21	23	26	30	26	23	28	33	28	25	28	40	22
12. Repeating rhythmically spoken syllables	127	85	81	155	125	121	148	96	146	122	102	120	103	129	132	144	109	121	159	78
13. Speaking as many words as possible within 2 minutes.	50	27	17	35	33	35	45	28	59	29	21	46	22	42	45	53	39	27	55	58
14. Lipreading with sound-perception and repeating.	65	31	32	46	47	49	51	28	62	63	71	65	35	47	51	71	32	54	72	22
15. Speaking correctly repeated words again.	100	68	81	97	94	97	99	59	100	86	81	91	78	93	97	100	81	93	100	62

Table 31

Group II. 8;0 – 8;11, N. 18, 8 boys – 10 girls. "Raw scores".

	21b.	22b.	23b.	24b.	25b.	26b.	27b.	28b.	29g.	30g.	31g.	32g.	33g.	34g.	35g.	36g.	37g.	38g.
1. Remembering simultaneously presented coloured rods.	15	15	16	14	14	15	15	14	16	15	15	15	15	16	15	14	13	15
2. Imitating shown successive folding movements.	5	8	4	6	8	3	7	7	8	5	6	7	7	5	7	7	6	7
3. Remembering simultaneously presented pictures.	9	9	11	9	10	10	9	9	10	9	8	9	9	10	9	9	8	9
4. Remembering successively presented pictures.	6	8	8	5	10	6	8	9	10	6	8	8	8	7	7	7	8	8
5. Repeating spoken series of digits.	5	6	3	3	6	0	5	6	6	3	6	6	6	3	5	5	7	6
6. Associating simultaneous digit-symbol.	24	34	27	17	25	33	23	27	37	24	19	29	27	31	28	34	25	30
7. Copying simultaneously presented geometrical figures from memory.	3	5	8	3	5	3	3	4	5	4	3	4	3	5	4	4	3	4
8. Identifying simultaneously presented geometrical figures from memory.	7	8	10	4	7	4	5	7	10	6	4	6	6	7	6	5	6	6
9. Tapping four cubes in a shown order.	7	11	5	9	12	5	9	10	12	5	9	11	9	6	11	11	9	11
10. Putting the fingers in a certain position according to an example.	14	14	11	12	14	10	14	13	14	13	11	14	15	11	15	14	16	15
11. Imitating shown finger-movements from memory.	32	33	23	28	32	27	35	30	37	27	29	32	35	25	36	33	41	37
12. Repeating rhythmically spoken syllables	120	139	97	113	139	98	125	162	128	103	154	125	137	105	145	141	152	146
13. Speaking as many words as possible within 2 minutes.	49	61	58	29	50	31	40	63	64	33	41	50	45	43	53	43	61	60
14. Lipreading with sound-perception and repeating.	55	80	38	63	78	45	87	77	72	48	88	68	73	50	68	73	87	79
15. Speaking correctly repeated words again.	83	98	59	86	100	76	100	98	99	79	100	99	99	74	98	97	100	97

Table 32

Group III. 9;0 – 9;11. N. 23, 14 boys – 9 girls. "Raw scores".

	39b.	40b.	41b.	42b.	43b.	44b.	45b.	46b.	47b.	48b.	49.b	50b.	51b.	15b.	53g.	54g.	55g.	56g.	57g.	58g.	59g.	60g.	61g.
1. Remembering simultaneously presented coloured rods.	15	16	15	15	16	15	14	16	15	17	15	16	15	15	14	14	15	16	14	14	16	15	14
2. Imitating shown successive folding movements.	7	6	7	7	6	5	6	9	7	8	7	7	6	6	7	8	6	7	7	6	7	7	7
3. Remembering simultaneously presented pictures.	9	10	9	9	11	10	9	10	10	10	10	10	8	8	9	10	8	9	9	10	9	9	9
4. Remembering successively presented pictures.	8	8	7	9	9	6	8	11	8	10	9	9	7	6	7	9	9	7	9	8	8	9	10
5. Repeating spoken series of digits.	5	6	5	5	6	3	5	6	5	6	6	6	5	5	3	7	5	5	7	5	6	6	7
6. Associating simultaneous digit-symbol.	28	34	31	29	37	31	26	45	30	32	28	34	36	26	21	36	36	29	28	28	40	28	25
7. Copying simultaneously presented geometrical figures from memory.	4	6	3	4	6	3	4	6	4	4	3	4	5	3	3	4	6	3	4	6	4	6	3
8. Identifying simultaneously presented geometrical figures from memory.	6	6	6	5	10	4	4	10	5	7	4	7	7	5	6	7	8	4	6	10	6	10	4
9. Tapping four cubes in a shown order.	11	10	9	10	9	8	6	12	11	12	9	11	9	8	8	11	9	4	10	10	10	10	10
10. Putting the fingers in a certain position according to an example.	15	12	14	15	13	11	14	16	14	12	15	15	12	14	14	15	11	14	15	13	15	16	
11. Imitating shown finger-movements from memory.	36	30	32	37	26	27	29	38	31	29	28	32	34	28	32	34	34	24	28	33	29	35	36
12. Repeating rhythmically spoken syllables	154	114	140	148	95	97	157	154	137	186	166	196	168	133	143	138	160	89	155	162	117	187	169
13. Speaking as many words as possible within 2 minutes.	70	45	48	42	65	59	40	62	48	53	42	67	51	42	93	66	70	47	60	67	56	39	
14. Lipreading with sound-perception and repeating.	85	61	73	72	61	59	81	83	74	82	84	86	80	69	70	79	87	58	76	83	69	73	85
15. Speaking correctly repeated words again.	98	83	100	96	89	79	98	100	91	95	96	100	97	78	92	90	100	84	96	100	85	95	100

Table 33
Group IV. 10;0 – 10;11, N. 22, 12 boys – 10 girls. "Raw scores".

	62b.	63b.	64b.	65b.	66b.	67b.	68b.	69b.	70b.	71b.	72.b	73b.	74.g.	75.g.	76.g.	77.g.	78.g.	79.g.	80.g.	81.g.	82.g.	83.g.
1. Remembering simultaneously presented coloured rods.	16	16	16	14	17	15	17	14	17	17	17	16	15	17	15	15	16	16	15	15	16	15
2. Imitating shown successive folding movements.	7	8	6	7	8	7	7	7	8	8	6	8	7	6	8	8	8	6	8	8	8	7
3. Remembering simultaneously presented pictures.	10	9	11	9	10	9	11	9	10	10	11	10	8	11	9	9	10	10	9	10	10	9
4. Remembering successively presented pictures.	9	10	10	9	12	10	10	10	10	12	11	12	10	12	11	12	9	9	10	10	11	11
5. Repeating spoken series of digits.	7	7	6	6	8	6	8	7	7	8	6	7	5	8	8	7	7	5	6	7	7	8
6. Associating simultaneous digit-symbol.	36	38	45	33	43	33	48	31	39	42	49	43	30	51	39	41	28	42	32	32	46	32
7. Copying simultaneously presented geometrical figures from memory.	5	4	10	4	10	4	9	3	4	5	10	4	3	10	4	3	6	5	3	6	6	4
8. Identifying simultaneously presented geometrical figures from memory.	7	7	10	6	10	8	10	7	7	6	10	8	7	10	6	6	6	9	4	6	9	7
9. Tapping four cubes in a shown order.	10	11	11	10	13	10	9	9	11	12	10	12	9	11	10	11	9	8	10	10	12	12
10. Putting the fingers in a certain position according to an example.	16	16	14	15	16	16	12	16	16	14	14	16	15	12	16	16	16	11	16	16	16	16
11. Imitating shown finger-movements from memory.	37	35	27	35	37	31	27	32	36	33	24	35	33	20	37	32	33	28	33	33	37	29
12. Repeating rhythmically spoken syllables	199	210	155	205	217	195	105	220	200	213	153	119	208	144	195	219	185	149	207	206	200	220
13. Speaking as many words as possible within 2 minutes.	69	70	75	59	72	49	80	40	73	73	70	75	47	77	61	65	68	67	70	60	81	56
14. Lipreading with sound-perception and repeating.	78	88	68	80	87	82	67	90	92	91	63	93	75	65	94	83	94	62	89	88	93	88
15. Speaking correctly repeated words again.	97	100	90	100	100	92	89	100	100	98	85	100	92	82	100	98	99	86	99	97	100	100

Total N.83

Table 34
CORRELATION-MATRIX of 15 selected variables.

	1 Si.C.	2 Su.Fo.	3 Si.Pi.	4 Su.Pi.	5 Di.Sp.	6 D.Sy.	7 Bt.C.	8 Bt.Id.	9 Knox	10 Bergès	11 Fi.Mov.	12 Rhythm	13 Or.Fl.	14 Lipr.	15 Spe. Rep.
1. Remembering simultaneously presented coloured rods.		+0.19	+0.81	+0.64	+0.46	+0.62	+0.70	+0.68	+0.31	+0.08	−0.03	+0.19	+0.60	+0.25	−0.13
2. Imitating shown successive folding movements.	+0.19		+0.03	+0.62	+0.68	+0.17	+0.04	+0.12	+0.75	+0.72	+0.67	+0.68	+0.49	+0.80	+0.79
3. Remembering simultaneously presented pictures.	+0.81	+0.03		+0.54	+0.39	+0.61	+0.78	+0.68	+0.20	−0.03	−0.15	−0.01	+0.50	+0.08	−0.30
4. Remembering successively presented pictures.	+0.64	+0.62	+0.54		+0.76	+0.54	+0.55	+0.56	+0.60	+0.52	+0.29	+0.63	+0.69	+0.63	+0.38
5. Repeating spoken series of digits.	+0.46	+0.68	+0.39	+0.76		+0.37	+0.41	+0.39	+0.64	+0.63	+0.50	+0.62	+0.67	+0.70	+0.51
6. Associating simultaneous digit-symbol.	+0.62	+0.17	+0.61	+0.54	+0.37		+0.63	+0.67	+0.35	+0.03	−0.06	+0.13	+0.51	+0.06	−0.08
7. Copying simultaneously presented geometrical figures from memory.	+0.70	+0.04	+0.78	+0.55	+0.41	+0.63		+0.79	+0.23	−0.03	−0.18	+0.01	+0.53	+0.03	−0.25
8. Identifying simultaneously presented geometrical figures from memory.	+0.68	+0.12	+0.68	+0.56	+0.39	+0.67	+0.79		+0.31	+0.03	−0.06	+0.02	+0.57	+0.05	−0.17
9. Tapping four cubes in a shown order.	+0.31	+0.75	+0.20	+0.60	+0.64	+0.35	+0.23	+0.31		+0.55	+0.52	+0.52	+0.55	+0.57	+0.59
10. Putting the fingers in a certain position according to an example.	+0.08	+0.72	−0.03	+0.52	+0.63	+0.03	−0.03	+0.03	+0.55		+0.82	+0.76	+0.43	+0.75	+0.72
11. Imitating shown fingermovements from memory.	−0.03	+0.67	−0.15	+0.29	+0.50	−0.06	−0.18	−0.06	+0.52	+0.82		+0.56	+0.30	+0.66	+0.72
12. Repeating rhythmically spoken syllables.	+0.19	+0.68	−0.01	+0.63	+0.62	+0.13	+0.01	+0.02	+0.52	+0.76	+0.56		+0.43	+0.76	+0.66
13. Speaking as many words as possible within 2 minutes.	+0.60	+0.49	+0.50	+0.69	+0.67	+0.51	+0.53	+0.57	+0.55	+0.43	+0.30	+0.43		+0.50	+0.32
14. Lipreading with sound-perception and repeating.	+0.25	+0.80	+0.08	+0.63	+0.70	+0.06	+0.03	+0.05	+0.57	+0.75	+0.66	+0.76	+0.50		+0.76
15. Speaking correctly repeated words again.	−0.13	+0.79	−0.30	+0.38	+0.51	−0.08	−0.25	−0.17	+0.59	+0.72	+0.72	+0.66	+0.32	+0.76	
Averages:	14.9	6.6	9.2	8.3	5.2	32.7	4.3	6.4	9.4	13.6	30.7	147.2	52.6	69.4	92.1

	1 Si.C.	2 Su.Fo.	3 Si.Pi.	4 Su.Pi	5 Di.Sp.	6 D.Sy.	7 Bt.C.	8 Bt.Id.	9 Knox	10 Bergès	11 Fi.Mov.	12 Rhythm	13 Or.Fl.	14 Lipr.	15 Spe. Rep.
1. Remembering simultaneously presented coloured rods.		−0.20	+0.83	+0.50	+0.26	+0.74	+0.73	+0.76	+0.12	−0.37	−0.34	−0.30	+0.30	−0.23	−0.50
2. Imitating shown successive folding movements.	−0.20		−0.20	+0.46	+0.53	−0.03	−0.23	−0.14	+0.81	+0.64	+0.63	+0.81	+0.63	+0.79	+0.73
3. Remembering simultaneously presented pictures.	+0.83	−0.20		+0.55	+0.39	+0.75	+0.89	+0.79	+0.08	−0.36	−0.25	−0.39	+0.30	−0.35	−0.62
4. Remembering successively presented pictures.	+0.50	+0.46	+0.55		+0.48	+0.45	+0.58	+0.60	+0.50	+0.08	+0.06	+0.21	+0.78	+0.18	+0.14
5. Repeating spoken series of digits.	+0.26	+0.53	+0.39	+0.48		+0.29	+0.37	+0.27	+0.62	+0.44	+0.50	+0.40	+0.62	+0.32	+0.23
6. Associating simultaneous digit-symbol.	+0.74	−0.03	+0.75	+0.45	+0.29		+0.60	+0.69	+0.21	−0.13	−0.00	−0.12	+0.29	−0.01	−0.26
7. Copying simultaneously presented geometrical figures from memory.	+0.73	−0.23	+0.89	+0.58	+0.37	+0.60		+0.81	+0.01	−0.32	−0.30	−0.50	+0.24	−0.35	−0.60
8. Identifying simultaneously presented geometrical figures from memory.	+0.76	−0.14	+0.79	+0.60	+0.27	+0.69	+0.81		+0.15	−0.20	−0.21	−0.33	+0.45	−0.21	−0.39
9. Tapping four cubes in a shown order.	+0.12	+0.81	+0.08	+0.50	+0.62	+0.21	+0.01	+0.15		+0.67	+0.58	+0.70	+0.66	+0.58	+0.54
10. Putting the fingers in a certain position according to an example.	−0.37	+0.64	−0.36	+0.08	+0.44	−0.13	−0.32	−0.20	+0.67		+0.90	+0.74	+0.34	+0.46	+0.71
11. Imitating shown finger-movements from memory.	−0.34	+0.63	−0.25	+0.06	+0.50	−0.00	−0.30	−0.21	+0.58	+0.90		+0.76	+0.30	+0.53	+0.65
12. Repeating rhythmically spoken syllables.	−0.30	+0.81	−0.39	+0.21	+0.40	−0.12	−0.50	−0.33	+0.70	+0.74	+0.76		+0.51	+0.67	+0.86
13. Speaking as many words as possible within 2 minutes.	+0.30	+0.63	+0.30	+0.78	+0.62	+0.29	+0.24	+0.45	+0.66	+0.34	+0.30	+0.51		+0.32	+0.40
14. Lipreading with sound-perception and repeating.	−0.23	+0.79	−0.35	+0.18	+0.32	−0.01	−0.35	−0.21	+0.58	+0.46	+0.53	+0.67	+0.32		+0.73
15. Speaking correctly repeated words again.	−0.50	+0.73	−0.62	+0.14	+0.23	−0.26	−0.60	−0.39	+0.54	+0.71	+0.65	+0.86	+0.40	+0.73	
Averages:	13.8	5.9	8.4	6.3	3.5	32.3	3.3	5.5	8.7	12.0	27.6	120.1	38.3	49.7	87.8
Standard deviations:	1.0	1.3	1.0	1.4	1.9	7.5	1.3	1.6	1.7	1.8	5.9	24.0	12.8	15.7	13.0

Table 36

CORRELATION-MATRIX of 15 selected variables.

Group II N.18

		1 Si.C.	2 Su.Fo.	3 Si.Pi.	4 Su.Pi.	5 Di.Sp.	6 D.Sy.	7 Bt.C.	8 Bt.Id.	9 Knox	10 Bergès	11 Fi.Mov.	12 Rhythm	13 Or.Fl.	14 Lipr.	15 Spe.Rep.
1.	Remembering simultaneously presented coloured rods.		−0.22	+0.58	+0.05	−0.32	+0.35	+0.49	+0.47	−0.31	−0.40	−0.39	−0.53	+0.02	−0.49	−0.46
2.	Imitating shown successive folding movements.	−0.22		−0.29	+0.63	+0.81	+0.17	−0.04	+0.18	+0.93	+0.68	+0.64	+0.69	+0.47	+0.76	+0.84
3.	Remembering simultaneously presented pictures.	+0.58	−0.29		+0.15	−0.52	+0.40	+0.75	+0.58	−0.30	−0.45	−0.52	−0.64	+0.06	−0.67	−0.65
4.	Remembering successively presented pictures.	+0.05	+0.63	+0.15		+0.65	+0.31	+0.36	+0.54	+0.58	+0.32	+0.38	+0.51	+0.70	+0.52	+0.48
5.	Repeating spoken series of digits.	−0.32	+0.81	−0.52	+0.65		−0.02	−0.10	+0.21	+0.76	+0.76	+0.72	+0.83	+0.66	+0.81	+0.79
6.	Associating simultaneous digit-symbol.	+0.35	+0.17	+0.40	+0.31	−0.02		+0.35	+0.46	+0.21	+0.11	+0.18	−0.04	+0.43	−0.12	+0.02
7.	Copying simultaneously presented geometrical figures from memory.	+0.49	−0.04	+0.75	+0.36	−0.10	+0.35		+0.79	−0.10	−0.23	−0.40	−0.30	+0.44	−0.41	−0.49
8.	Identifying simultaneously presented geometrical figures from memory.	+0.47	+0.18	+0.58	+0.54	+0.21	+0.46	+0.79		+0.07	+0.12	−0.01	−0.11	+0.72	−0.22	−0.24
9.	Tapping four cubes in a shown order.	−0.31	+0.93	−0.30	+0.58	+0.76	+0.21	−0.10	+0.07		+0.64	+0.68	+0.74	+0.48	+0.76	+0.86
10.	Putting the fingers in a certain position according to an example.	−0.40	+0.68	−0.45	+0.32	+0.76	+0.11	−0.23	+0.12	+0.64		+0.89	+0.58	+0.50	+0.58	+0.68
11.	imitating shown finger-movements from memory.	−0.39	+0.64	−0.52	+0.38	+0.72	+0.18	−0.40	−0.01	+0.68	+0.89		+0.66	+0.48	+0.73	+0.79
12.	Repeating rhythmically spoken syllables.	−0.53	+0.69	−0.64	+0.51	+0.83	−0.04	−0.30	−0.11	+0.74	+0.66	+0.66		+0.52	+0.86	+0.84
13.	Speaking as many words as possible within 2 minutes.	+0.02	+0.47	+0.06	+0.70	+0.66	+0.43	+0.44	+0.72	+0.48	+0.50	+0.48	+0.52		+0.34	+0.29
14.	Lipreading with sound-perception and repeating.	−0.49	+0.76	−0.67	+0.52	+0.81	−0.12	−0.41	−0.22	+0.76	+0.50	+0.73	+0.86	+0.34		+0.92
15.	Speaking correctly repeated words again.	−0.46	+0.84	−0.65	+0.48	+0.79	+0.02	−0.49	−0.24	+0.86	+0.58	+0.79	+0.84	+0.29	+0.92	
	Averages:	14.8	6.3	9.2	7.6	4.8	27.4	4.1	6.3	9.0	13.3	31.8	129.4	48.6	68.3	91.2
	Standard deviations:	0.8	1.4	0.7	0.7	1.8	5.2	1.3	1.7	2.4	1.7	4.7	20.0	11.2	15.3	12.1

	1 Si.C.	2 Su.Fo.	3 Si.Pi.	4 Su.Pi.	5 Di.Sp.	6 D.Sy.	7 Bt.C.	8 Bt.Id.	9 Knox	10 Bergès	11 Fi.Mov.	12 Rhythm	13 Or.Fl.	14 Lipr.	15 Spe. Rep.
1. Remembering simultaneously presented coloured rods.		+0.15	+0.76	+0.44	+0.16	+0.71	+0.66	+0.67	+0.53	−0.47	−0.24	−0.15	+0.23	−0.25	−0.24
2. Imitating shown successive folding movements.	+0.15		−0.12	+0.66	+0.38	+0.18	−0.05	+0.21	+0.47	+0.56	+0.63	+0.63	−0.08	+0.72	+0.71
3. Remembering simultaneously presented pictures.	+0.76	−0.12		+0.36	+0.23	+0.68	+0.63	+0.53	+0.34	−0.44	−0.38	−0.30	+0.05	−0.32	−0.35
4. Remembering successively presented pictures.	+0.44	+0.66	+0.36		+0.61	+0.35	+0.38	+0.39	+0.55	+0.26	+0.33	+0.38	−0.05	+0.42	+0.47
5. Repeating spoken series of digits.	+0.16	+0.38	+0.23	+0.61			+0.32	+0.28	+0.36	+0.18	+0.21	+0.34	+0.08	+0.33	+0.35
6. Associating simultaneous digit-symbol.	+0.71	+0.18	+0.68	+0.35			+0.77	+0.80	+0.32	−0.25	−0.11	−0.26	+0.32	−0.21	−0.19
7. Copying simultaneously presented geometrical figures from memory.	+0.66	−0.05	+0.63	+0.38	+0.32	+0.77		+0.80	+0.27	−0.49	−0.21	+0.24	−0.10	+0.24	+0.22
8. Identifying simultaneously presented geometrical figures from memory.	+0.67	+0.21	+0.53	+0.39	+0.28	+0.80	+0.80		+0.41	−0.32	−0.05	+0.24	−0.14	−0.17	−0.14
9. Tapping four cubes in a shown order.	+0.53	+0.47	+0.34	+0.55	+0.36	+0.32	+0.27	+0.41		+0.20	+0.47	+0.24	+0.38	+0.24	+0.22
10. Putting the fingers in a certain position according to an example.	−0.47	+0.56	−0.44	+0.26	+0.18	−0.25	−0.49	−0.32	+0.20		+0.82	+0.69	−0.10	−0.04	+0.76
11. Imitating shown fingermovements from memory.	−0.24	+0.63	−0.38	+0.33	+0.21	−0.11	−0.21	−0.05	+0.47	+0.82		+0.56	−0.04	+0.59	+0.63
12. Repeating rhythmically spoken syllables.	−0.15	+0.63	−0.30	+0.38	+0.34	−0.26	+0.24	+0.24	+0.24	+0.69	+0.56		−0.14	+0.85	+0.75
13. Speaking as many words as possible within 2 minutes.	+0.23	−0.08	+0.05	−0.05	+0.08	+0.32	−0.10	−0.14	+0.38	−0.10	−0.04	−0.14		−0.15	−0.01
14. Lipreading with sound-perception and repeating.	−0.25	+0.72	−0.32	+0.42	+0.33	−0.21	+0.24	−0.17	+0.24	−0.04	+0.59	+0.85	−0.15		+0.82
15. Speaking correctly repeated words again.	−0.24	+0.71	−0.35	+0.47	+0.35	−0.19	+0.22	−0.14	+0.22	+0.76	+0.63	+0.75	−0.01	+0.82	
Averages:	15.1	6.8	9.4	8.3	5.5	31.6	4.2	6.3	9.4	13.9	31.3	46.3	55.0	75.2	93.1
Standard deviations:	0.8	0.9	0.8	1.3	1.0	5.5	1.1	1.9	1.8	1.5	3.7	29.0	13.9	9.2	7.0

Group IV N.22

Table 38

CORRELATION-MATRIX of 15 selected variables.

		1 Si.C.	2 Su.Fo.	3 Si.Pi.	4 Su.Pi	5 Di.Sp.	6 D.Sy.	7 Bt.C.	8 Bt.Id.	9 Knox	10 Berges	11 Fi.Mov.	12 Rhythm	13 Or.Fl.	14 Lipr.	15 Spe. Rep.
1.	Remembering simultaneously presented coloured rods.		−0.09	+0.75	+0.38	+0.33	+0.72	+0.67	+0.58	+0.32	−0.43	−0.27	−0.48	+0.77	−0.28	−0.39
2.	Imitating shown successive folding movements.	−0.09		−0.38	+0.14	+0.39	−0.32	−0.45	−0.59	+0.38	+0.69	+0.78	+0.46	+0.09	+0.89	+0.83
3.	Remembering simultaneously presented pictures.	+0.75	−0.38		+0.21	+0.26	+0.74	+0.84	+0.67	+0.12	−0.54	−0.51	−0.69	+0.72	−0.46	−0.53
4.	Remembering successively presented pictures.	+0.38	+0.14	+0.21		+0.48	+0.57	+0.29	+0.27	+0.68	+0.01	−0.19	−0.07	+0.28	+0.08	−0.06
5.	Repeating spoken series of digits.	+0.33	+0.39	+0.26	+0.48		+0.26	+0.23	+0.05	+0.54	+0.13	+0.08	+0.04	+0.31	+0.38	+0.30
6.	Associating simultaneous digit-symbol.	+0.72	−0.32	+0.74	+0.57	+0.26		+0.69	+0.75	+0.34	−0.57	−0.44	−0.62	+0.73	−0.48	−0.52
7.	Copying simultaneously presented geometrical figures from memory.	+0.67	−0.45	+0.84	+0.29	+0.23	+0.69		+0.79	+0.19	−0.50	−0.54	−0.52	+0.55	−0.55	−0.59
8.	Identifying simultaneously presented geometrical figures from memory.	+0.58	−0.59	+0.67	+0.27	+0.05	+0.75	+0.79		+0.14	−0.55	−0.51	−0.61	+0.38	−0.63	−0.64
9.	Tapping four cubes in a shown order.	+0.32	+0.38	+0.12	+0.68	+0.54	+0.34	+0.19	+0.14		+0.35	+0.23	+0.21	+0.40	+0.40	+0.38
10.	Putting the fingers in a certain position according to an example.	−0.43	+0.69	−0.54	+0.01	+0.13	−0.57	−0.50	−0.55	+0.35		+0.73	+0.67	−0.32	+0.82	+0.83
11.	Imitating shown fingermovements from memory.	−0.27	+0.78	−0.51	−0.19	+0.08	−0.44	−0.54	−0.51	+0.23	+0.73		+0.55	−0.10	+0.77	+0.86
12.	Repeating rhythmically spoken syllables.	−0.48	+0.46	−0.69	−0.07	+0.04	−0.62	−0.52	−0.61	+0.21	+0.67	+0.55		−0.50	+0.57	+0.63
13.	Speaking as many words as possible within 2 minutes.	+0.77	+0.09	+0.72	+0.28	+0.31	+0.73	+0.55	+0.38	+0.40	+0.82	+0.77	+0.57		−0.14	+0.92
14.	Lipreading with sound-perception and repeating.	−0.28	+0.89	−0.46	+0.08	+0.38	−0.48	−0.55	−0.63	+0.40	+0.82	+0.77	+0.57	−0.14		+0.92
15.	Speaking correctly repeated words again.	−0.39	+0.83	−0.53	−0.06	+0.30	−0.52	−0.59	−0.64	+0.38	+0.83	+0.86	+0.63	−0.16	+0.92	
	Averages:	15.8	7.3	9.7	10.5	6.9	38.8	5.5	7.5	10.5	15.0	32.0	187.5	66.2	82.3	95.6

Table 39: We give the averages with their standard-deviations per group and of the total:

Table 39
The averages per age-group in the 15 tests. "Raw scores".

	1 Si.C.	2 Su.Fo.	3 Si.Pi.	4 Su.Pi	5 Di.Sp.	6 D.Sy.	7 Bt.C.	8 Bt.Id.	9 Knox	10 Bergès	11 Fi.Mov.	12 Rhytm	13 Or.Fl.	14 Lipr.	15 Spe. Rep.
Group 7;0 – 7;11 N.29	13.8 ±1.0	5.9 ±1.3	8.4 ±1.0	6.3 ±1.4	3.5 ±1.9	32.3 ±7.5	3.3 ±1.3	5.5 ±1.6	8.7 ±1.7	12.0 ±1.8	27.6 ±5.9	120.1 ±24.0	38.3 ±12.8	49.7 ±15.7	87.8% ±13.0%
Group 8;0 – 8;11 N.18	14.8 ±0.8	6.3 ±1.4	9.2 ±0.7	7.6 ±1.3	4.8 ±1.8	27.4 ±5.2	4.1 ±1.3	6.3 ±1.7	9.0 ±2.4	13.3 ±1.7	31.8 ±4.7	129.4 ±20.0	48.6 ±11.2	68.3 ±15.3	91.2% ±12.1%
Group 9;0 – 9;11 N. 23	15.1 ±0.8	6.8 ±0.9	9.4 ±0.8	8.3 ±1.3	5.5 ±1.0	31.6 ±5.5	4.2 ±1.1	6.3 ±1.9	9.4 ±1.8	13.9 ±1.5	31.3 ±3.7	145.3 ±29.0	55.0 ±13.9	75.2 ±9.2	93.1% ±7.0%
Group 10;0 – 10;11 N.22	15.8 ±1.0	7.3 ±0.8	9.7 ±0.8	10.5 ±1.1	6.9 ±0.9	38.8 ±6.8	5.5 ±2.5	7.5 ±1.7	10.5 ±1.3	15.0 ±1.6	32.0 ±4.5	187.5 ±39.0	66.2 ±10.8	82.3 ±10.9	95.6% ±5.8%
All the children N.83	14.9 ±1.1	6.6 ±1.2	9.2 ±1.0	8.3 ±2.0	5.2 ±1.9	32.7 ±7.4	4.3 ±1.8	6.4 ±1.9	9.4 ±1.9	13.6 ±1.9	30.7 ±5.0	147.2 ±37.7	52.6 ±15.8	69.4 ±17.5	92.1% ±10.0%
Maximum:	19	9	16	16	17	57	10	10	15	16	42	210	±90	100	100%

6. A THREE FACTORS' ANALYSIS

On the face of it the tests used can be divided into four categories:
"supple use of the mouth when speaking" in tests (5), (13), (14) and (15);
"fluent, fine motor function" in tests (10), (11) and (12);
"memory for successively presented visual data" in tests (2), (4) and (9);
and "memory for simultaneously presented visual data" in tests (1), (3), (6), (7) and (8).

Because the first three categories seemed to be involved most of all in speech, their scores were totalled and product-moment correlations of these sum totals were worked out per group. The quotients found are put together in Table 40 in a matrix, the four age-groups consecutively in each cell.

Table 40.

	"Fluent fine motor function"	"Memory for successively presented visual data"
"supple use of the mouth when speaking"	(0.88) (0.83) (0.61) (0.32)	(0.65) (0.79) (0.60) (0.65)
"Fluent fine motor function"		(0.74) (0.68) (0.48) (0.14)

Thus the correlations dropped off with age, except those of "supple use of mouth when speaking" with "memory for successively presented visual data". This prompted our mathematical advisor Van der Sanden (1974), to whom we presented the test results obtained, to choose a certain type of factor analysis.

A verbatim account of Van der Sanden's advice:
"In the tables 30-38 the reader sees a survey of the 15 tests which were given to the children, plus their results, as well as of the product-moment correlation-matrices per group. The question is: which factors have been most determining in the results of these tests and are there any differences between the four age-groups as regards the importance of these factors?

For this question the matrices mentioned were subjected to an INDSCAL-analysis. This method was originally developed by Carrol and Chang (1970) in order to analyse individual differences between similarity-opinions in the multi-dimensional scaling of the stimuli

116

judged (INDSCAL = INdividual Differences SCALing). Van der Sanden (1973) showed how this method can be applied for the simultaneous analysis of correlation-matrices obtained from different groups of subjects on separate occasions. What is special about this method is that several matrices of similarity-measures (in this case correlations) can be analysed at the same time. By means of this both the similarities and the differences between the matrices come to the fore.

When we write down the correlation between two tests (j and k) for a certain group of children (t) as $r_{jk}^{(t)}$, then according to the INDSCAL model.

Figure 30.

$$r_{jk}^{(t)} = \sum_{p=1}^{m} w_{tp} x_{jp} x_{kp}$$

where m is the number of dimensions (factors) of the space in which the tests can be represented. These m dimensions are the factors in our problem which we want to trace.

The quantities x_{jp} and x_{kp} are the co-ordinates of the tests j and k on dimension (factor) p; they are constant for all the correlation-matrices (read: groups), included in the analysis. One could call them the factor-loadings, though the analogy with the "classic" factor-analysis does not quite hold.

The variable w_{tp} is the weight (read: importance) of factor p to group t. Consequently these weights may differ for each group and can therefore provide us with information on differences in functioning between the age-groups.

It proved best to start from three factors. The 4-factor solution was not usable because on the fourth factor one of the age-groups appeared to have a negative weight, which is in conflict with the INDSCAL-model. The correlation between observed and predicted data in a 3-factor analysis was: 0.94". (Conclusion of Van der Sanden's report).

Factor 1: eupraxia versus simultaneous visual cognition
The loadings of the 15 variables are given in a scheme, see Figure 31.

This first factor can be interpreted as follows: It is a *polar* factor.

In the plus-loadings one can find those tests which relate to the fine *motor* function of fingers and mouth. It seems that eupraxia of finger-movements goes with eupraxia of oral movement. Among children who controlled their finger-movements well, the speech-movements were

117

Figure 31

3-Factor analysis

(10) Putting the fingers in a certain
position according to an example.   + 0.350
(14) Lipreading with sound-perception and
repeating.   + 0.323
(15) Speaking correctly repeated words
again.   + 0.318
(12) Repeating rhythmically spoken
syllables.   + 0.304
(11) Imitating shown finger-movements
from memory   + 0.293
(2) Imitating seen successive folding
movements.   + 0.274
(4) Remembering successively presented
pictures.   − 0.028
(9) Tapping four cubes in a shown order.   − 0.033

(5) Repeating spoken series of digits.   − 0.053

(1) Remembering simultaneously
presented coloured rods.   − 0.196
(13) Speaking as many words as possible
within 2 minutes.   − 0.239
(3) Remembering simultaneously
presented pictures.   − 0.245
(8) Identifying simultaneously presented
geometrical figures from memory.   − 0.287
(7) Copying simultaneously presented
geometrical figures from memory.   − 0.287
(6) Simultaneous digit/symbol
association.   − 0.304

Importance of this factor, deduced from
the weights to the four age-groups:

7 years olds 3.991
8 years olds 2.700
9 years olds 4.590

Factor I   Scheme of the loadings in steps of 5.

Rank:

Importance of this factor to the 4 age-groups:

118

co-ordinated well too, and conversely those with clumsy fingermovements were "clumsy" speakers. – This eupraxia is also related to rhythmic movement, which points to a common factor.

In the minus-loadings all the tests concerned with the memory for *simultaneously* presented *visual* data are concentrated in a pattern. From the polarity of factor I it appears that those who were less fluent in their motor function did better in tests which were related to the memory for simultaneously presented visual data and vice versa.

Between both poles there are three tests which are concerned with the memory for *successively* presented visual data; they both fall outside the loadings. These tests are not concerned so much with fine articulation. When repeating digits it is not a question of fine articulation; it is sufficient that the experimenter knows which digit the child means.

The test of "being able to say as many words as possible within 2 minutes" demands speech and yet it lies within the circle of the tests which relate to memory for simultaneously presented visual data. According to factor I this test measures something which corresponds with this, which can be explained from the *written form* of the words being a simultaneously presented visual datum (see below NB.). Here too it is not a matter of fine articulation but it is sufficient for the experimenter to understand what the child means. It matters little whether the words were remembered motorily or visually. Obviously the children have remembered the words visually and "translated" them into speech.

There are memory-tests in which the visually presented figure is more easily named, and others in which it is less easily named. For example, the colours and pictures of the tests concerned are easily named, the geometrical figures and nonsense symbols are not. In factor I the latter are farthest away from the tests which relate to the speech motor function.

The *importance* of this factor increases with age. In the group of 7-year olds and even more in that of 8-year olds, those whose motor function was less fluent were at a disadvantage, because they also achieved less as regards the memory for simultaneous data.

The older children, 9 and 10 years of age, those who reacted less fluently motorily, appeared to make better use of their memory for these data.

NB. We have composed *a test of non-pictorial* (i.e. non-imaginative) *words* (van Uden, 1977, e.g. too, yet, nor, by etc., altogether 18 of them). The test has to be applied in the same way as Hiskey's Test "Visual Attention Span" (3), but instead of pictures, non-imaginative words are used. Miss Lieve Merken, psychological associate, has applied this test and compared its results with those of the "Visual Attention Span", "memory for colours", and Benton's Test, on our request. She found significant correlations, from which it can be predicted whether a child may develop a good memory for the written form of words or not (Merken, 1978).

Factor II: active versus passive
The loadings of the 15 variables are given in a scheme, see Figure 32.

This factor can be interpreted as follows:
Again it is a *polar* function.
The plus-loadings concern all the tests which demand more activity from the child.
In the minus-loadings there are the two memory-tests for simultaneously presented colours and pictures, which require the least activity and in which the child can position himself passively, saturate himself with the data and remember them in that way (cf. Hofmarksrichter, 1931; Oléron, 1953).
In between we find three tests which do not load on factor II. Two of these concern the memory for simultaneously presented geometrical figures, which have to be drawn and identified, and one ditto for non-sense-symbols; one can call them neither mainly active nor mainly passive.
It may be remarkable that the test in which successively presented pictures have to be remembered belongs to the tests which require activities. This does not seem to be in conflict with the interpretation of this factor: remembering successively presented visual material requires more activity than remembering this same material simultaneously presented.
Among the 10 positively loaded tests of factor II are all those which directly concern speech-training; this indeed requires rather a lot of activity from deaf children.
The polarity of factor II means that children who achieved less where activity was required, achieved more where they could saturate themselves passively with visual impressions.
The *importance* of factor II decreases with age, in contrast with factor I. This means that the difference between children who were not particularly active but who reached better results in the passive memory-tasks and others who were more active and achieved less passively, decreased with age. As regards factor II the groups become more homogeneous.
The group of the 8-year olds, who showed a somewhat variant picture in factor I, show, as regards the importance of factor II, rather a sharp increase. In this group, which had to be selected less strictly according to the criteria, a greater number of less homogeneous children was present than in the other groups. Besides, this group was the smallest.

Factor III: a "forget-factor".
The loadings of the 15 variables are given in a scheme, see Figure 33.
I owe the interpretation of this factor to Van der Sanden (1974). All

3-Factor analysis

Factor II Scheme of the loadings in steps of 5.

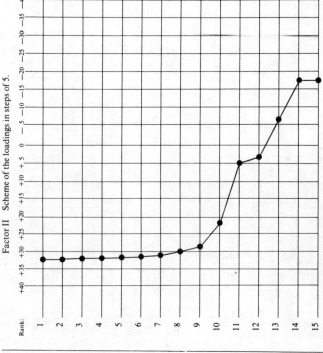

(12) Repeating rhythmically spoken syllables. +0.328

(10) Putting the fingers in a certain position according to an example. +0.324

(15) Speaking correctly repeated words again. +0.318

(5) Repeating spoken series of digits. +0.317

(13) Speaking as many words as possible within 2 minutes. +0.315

(11) Imitating shown finger-movements from memory +0.314

(2) Imitating seen successive folding movements. +0.305

(9) Tapping four cubes in a shown order. +0.302

(14) Lipreading with sound-perception and repeating. +0.293

(4) Remembering successively presented pictures. +0.220

(8) Identifying simultaneously presented geometrical figures from memory. +0.050

(6) Simultaneous digit/symbol association. +0.030

(7) Copying simultaneously presented geometrical figures from memory. — 0.068

(3) Remembering simultaneously presented pictures. — 0.174

(1) Remembering simultaneously presented coloured rods. — 0.174

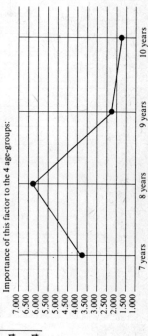

Importance of this factor to the 4 age-groups:

Importance of this factor, deduced from the weights to the four age-groups:

7 years olds 3.87162
8 years olds 6.11563
9 years olds 2.26402
10 years olds 1.54090

Figure 33

3-Factor analysis

(1) Remembering simultaneously presented coloured rods. — 0.410

(9) Tapping four cubes in a shown order. — 0.383

(4) Remembering successively presented pictures. — 0.367

(2) Imitating seen successive folding movements. — 0.316

(3) Remembering simultaneously presented pictures. — 0.304

(6) Simultaneous digit/symbol association. — 0.303

(5) Repeating spoken series of digits. — 0.285

(7) Copying simultaneously presented geometrical figures from memory. — 0.230

(8) Identifying simultaneously presented geometrical figures from memory. — 0.200

(14) Lipreading with sound-perception and repeating. — 0.193

(15) Speaking correctly repeated words again. — 0.144

(11) Imitating shown finger-movements from memory — 0.127

(12) Repeating rhythmically spoken syllables. — 0.091

(13) Speaking as many words as possible within 2 minutes. — 0.082

(10) Putting the fingers in a certain position according to an example — 0.060

Importance of this factor, deduced from the weights to the four age-groups:

7 years olds 3.51918
8 years olds 2.23782

122

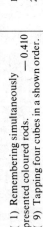

Factor III   Scheme of the loadings in steps of 5.

Rank:
1
2
3
4
5
6
7
8
9
10
11
12
13
14
15

+40 +35 +30 +25 +20 +15 +10 +5 0 −5 −10 −15 −20 −25 −30 −35 −40

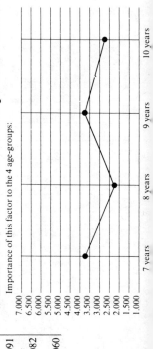

Importance of this factor to the 4 age-groups:

7.000
6.500
6.000
5.500
5.000
4.500
4.000
3.500
3.000
2.500
2.000
1.500
1.000

7 years   8 years   9 years   10 years

the loadings are negative. The more "important" this factor is to certain children, the less will they achieve in the tests which load this factor. As all the tests concerned relate to the memory, this achievement of less means forgetting. This "forget-factor" appears to be nearly equally "important" to all the age-groups.

It is not a polar factor. That which lay apart in the two other factors, i.e. memory for simultaneously and successively presented data, goes together here. The loadings decrease continuously.

It is remarkable that the 10 tests which load factor III all involve remembering ad hoc. The remaining five concern routine-tasks which the children perform all day through, or tasks which do not relate to the memory.

7. DISCUSSION

a. Comments on some of the tests used and their validity

"Intransitive movements"
Ad (10) "Putting the fingers in a certain position according to an example", test by Bergès and Lézine (1963). We have already mentioned the distinction by Kaplan (1972, see Brown, 1972) between transitive and intransitive movements.

This test and that of van Uden (11) concern an eupraxia of the fingers for intransitive movements. We chose these ones because we had nothing to go by for a diagnosis of the backgrounds of speech difficulties, when using tests with transitive movements, such as building, dressing oneself etc. Only heavily dyspraxic or apraxic children could be detected in the latter way.

Control of the "body-scheme"
The tests by Bergès and Lézine and van Uden actually are tests of the control of the "body-scheme", including a programming of the motor brain and a "gnosis", i.e. a recognition of the positions of the limbs: above – below, at right – at left, in front – behind. The tests include a second part, namely one with positions for arms and hands, concerning the coarser motor function, a control of the "body-scheme". In 24 children aged between 5 and 7 years, we found a correlation of .52 (p < 0.01) between this "body-part" of the tests and their "finger-part". But we found only a low correlation of this second part (.47 p < 0.05), and a high correlation (.79 p < 0.001) of the "finger-part", with our "Lipreading with sound perception and repeating"-test (14). All this was, however, also connected with a more refined scoring. With our rhythm-test (12): .71 (p < 0.001) we found a similar correlation.

Eurhythmia

Ad (12) "Repeating rhythmically spoken syllables". Seashore (1937), Wing (1968), Stambak (1965), Birch and Belmont (1965), Kahn and Birch (1968) constructed rhythm-tests without speech, amongst other things by *tapping* on a table. Because our diagnosis for deaf children concerned speech-training, we constructed a rhythm-test with "baba"-syllables.

On 92 children the rhythmic patterns of the syllable-test were also used for imitating tapping a rhythm on a table. The results showed a correlation of .82 between "tap"-rhythm and "baba"-rhythm. Further, seven teachers were asked for their opinion on their children's rhythmic moving and ability to *dance* by comparing them in pairs. The following correlations with the "baba"-rhythm were found: 0.56, 0.74, 0.83, 0.28, 0.70, 0.49 and 0.62 respectively. The second, third and fifth were significant ($p < 0.05$). The teacher in rhythmics was also asked to give an opinion on 37 children by comparing them in pairs. The correlation with that opinion was 0.62 ($p < 0.001$).

"Eupraxia-inventories"

The validity of the three tests on motor function has been examined by us with the help of a "eupraxia-inventory".

Through observation we collected many details of children's behaviours, especially of infants, which behaviours were concerned with "eupraxia in daily life", mainly transitive movements.

The house-parents of the residence were asked to fill in the inventories. We compared the results of the *2nd inventory* with the total results of our three tests ("fluent fine motor function"), and found the following correlations in 8 groups of children: .55, .65, .54, .66, .37, .42, .46 and .58. The first, second and eight correlations are significant ($p < 0.05$).

The *1st inventory* for preschool children is used routinely for diagnostic purposes, especially to find out whether the child concerned is suffering from the "syndrome of dyspraxia". All children have been investigated at least twice, most of them three times from $3^1/_2$-$6^1/_2$ years of age (cf. van Uden, 1980). – In 95 children of 5;7-6;5 years of age (last investigation) we found these correlations in Table 43. See p. 133.

I *Inventory for eupraxia of prelingually profoundly deaf children of 3¹/₂-7 years of age.*

Name: ....   Born: ....
Examination date: ....
Age: ....
Examiner(s): ....
Total score (max. 35)   ....
Developmental age: ....

N.B.
a. Are there any anatomical abnormalities in legs, feet, arms, hands?

b. Is the child wearing arch supports?

c. Is the child athetoid, or spastic?

athetoid
{
0 = not disturbed
1 = slightly disturbed
2 = moderately disturbed
3 = severely disturbed
4 = very severely disturbed
}

spastic
{
0 = not disturbed
1 = slightly disturbed
2 = moderately disturbed
3 = severely disturbed
4 = very severely disturbed
}

Behaviour:
Circle the correct answer

1. Can climb stairs:	has to be helped 0	foot by foot ¹/₂	reasonably quick 1
2. Can come down the stairs:	has to be helped 0	foot by foot ¹/₂	reasonably quick 1
3. Can hop:	not at all 0	clumsily ¹/₂	well 1
4. Holds writing or drawing material very loosely or clumsily:	remarkably often 0	sometimes ¹/₂	no trouble 1
5. Movements are slightly jerky:	remarkably often 0	sometimes ¹/₂	seldom or never 1
6. Can handle scissors:	remarkably badly 0	moderately well ¹/₂	no trouble 1
7. Knocks things over:	remarkably often 0	sometimes ¹/₂	seldom or never 1

8.	Movements are spasmodic:	seldom or never 1	sometimes $1/2$	remarkably often 0
9.	Is clumsy when dressing himself (e.g. uses wrong sleeve, confuses front with back, left with right, etc.):	seldom or never 1	sometimes $1/2$	remarkably often 0
10.	Trips:	seldom or never 1	sometimes $1/2$	remarkably often 0
11.	Forgets where he/she put things (loses things):	seldom or never 1	sometimes $1/2$	remarkably often 0
12.	Walks into things:	seldom or never 1	sometimes $1/2$	remarkably often 0
13.	Can tie a knot (e.g. in shoelace):	no trouble 1	fairly well $1/2$	not at all 0
14.	Can undo and do up zip of his/her jacket:	no trouble 1	fairly well $1/2$	not at all 0
15.	Seems to have difficulties in balancing (e.g. on the stairs, on a scooter, possibly even when walking etc.):	seldom or never 1	sometimes $1/2$	remarkably often 0
16.	Can tie a bow:	no trouble 1	fairly well $1/2$	not at all 0
17.	Walks stiffly (e.g. taking small steps):	seldom or never 1	sometimes $1/2$	nearly always 0
18.	Can button up his/her coat:	no trouble 1	fairly well $1/2$	not at all 0
19.	Can blow his/her nose:	no trouble 1	clumsily $1/2$	not at all 0
20.	His/her whole manner is clumsy, awkward:	seldom or never 1	sometimes $1/2$	remarkably often 0
21.	Walks with his/her feet turned out:	seldom or never 1	sometimes $1/2$	remarkably often 0
22.	Puts shoes on the wrong feet:	seldom or never 1	sometimes $1/2$	remarkably often 0
23.	Is clumsy when washing him/herself:	seldom or never 1	sometimes $1/2$	remarkably often 0

24.	Walks with his/her feet turned inwards:	remarkably often 0	sometimes $1/2$	seldom or never 1
25.	Bumps into other children:	remarkably often 0	sometimes $1/2$	seldom or never 1
26.	Puts gloves on wrong hand:	remarkably often 0	sometimes $1/2$	seldom or never 1
27.	Drags one of his feet when walking:	nearly always 0	sometimes $1/2$	seldom or never 1
28.	Often drops things:	remarkably often 0	sometimes $1/2$	seldom or never 1
29.	Always walks as if he/she is going to fall forward:	nearly always 0	sometimes $1/2$	seldom or never 1
30.	Can catch ball:	seldom or never 0	sometimes $1/2$	no trouble
31.	Walks on toes instead of on the whole foot:	nearly always 0	sometimes $1/2$	seldom or never 1
32.	Spills his food:	remarkably often 0	sometimes $1/2$	seldom or never 1
33.	Walks with legs apart:	nearly always 0	sometimes $1/2$	seldom or never 1
34.	Can blow:	not at all 0	fairly well $1/2$	no trouble
35.	Handles cutlery clumsily (e.g. does not hold spoon straight or turns it upside down, holds fork against the cheeck, etc.)	remarkably often 0	sometimes $1/2$	seldom or never 1

Total: _____ + _____

Total: _____

127

Table 41.
Standardisation of the Inventory for eupraxic behaviour of prelingually profoundly deaf children, 3½-7 years of age (max. 35)

Age	Number of children involved	Average scores
3;6 - 4;0	11	20 ± 7
4;1 - 4;5	14	22 ± 5
4;6 - 5;0	20	24 ± 6
5;1 - 5;5	23	27 ± 7
5;6 - 6;0	22	29 ± 5
6;1 - 6;5	19	30 ± 4

Figure 34

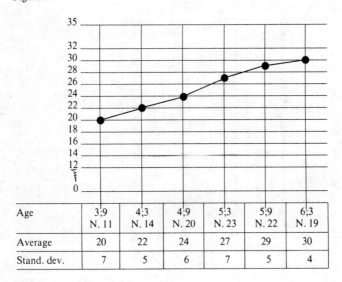

Age	3;9 N. 11	4;3 N. 14	4;9 N. 20	5;3 N. 23	5;9 N. 22	6;3 N. 19
Average	20	22	24	27	29	30
Stand. dev.	7	5	6	7	5	4

128

II. *Inventory for eupraxia of prelingually profoundly deaf children aged from 7 to 10.*

Name: .... Born: ....
Examination date: ....
Age: ....
Examiner(s): ....
Total score (max. 40): ....
Developmental age: ....

N.B.

a. Are there any anatomical abnormalities in legs, feet, arms, hands?
....

b. Is the child wearing arch supports?
....

c. Is the child athetoid, or spastic?

Athetoid
{
0: not disturbed
1: slightly disturbed
2: moderately disturbed
3: severely disturbed
4: very severely disturbed
}

Spastic
{
0: not disturbed
1: slightly disturbed
2: moderately disturbed
3: severely disturbed
4: very severely disturbed
}

Behaviour:
Circle the appropriate answer:

1. Can the child hop, dance, jump, run etc.?
   - Practically unable to 0
   - clumsily $1/2$
   - very capably 1

2. Does the child have difficulty in finding the correct words even though he knows them very well?
   - often 0
   - sometimes $1/2$
   - seldom or never 1

3. Does the child shuffle when walking?
   - often 0
   - sometimes $1/2$
   - seldom or never 1

4. Does the child walk as if about to fall forward?
   - very much 0
   - moderately $1/2$
   - normally 1

5. When the child leaves the room or the class, does he leave the door (perhaps door and window facing each other) open?
   - often 0
   - sometimes $1/2$
   - seldom or never 1

6. Does the child show spasmodic movements?
   - very strongly 0
   - moderately $1/2$
   - practically none 1

7. When the child has to step over something, does he do this clumsily, for example by not lifting his leg high enough, so that he (nearly) trips, etc.?
   - often 0
   - sometimes $1/2$
   - seldom or never 1

129

8. Does the child seem to have difficulty in balancing (for example on the bike, or simply walking)?	often 0	sometimes ½	seldom or never 1
9. When you ask the child for example to set the table, to lay his clothes ready, to pack a suit-case, does he forget parts of the instructions?	often 0	sometimes ½	seldom or never 1
10. Does the child experience difficulties with the order in writing, of letters, of words, or numbers?	often 0	sometimes ½	seldom or never 1
11. Is the child's whole manner of behaviour clumsy, awkward?	often 0	sometimes ½	seldom or never 1
12. Is the child's behaviour rhythmic in the "Music-and-Movement" lessons?	seldom or never 0	sometimes ½	often 1
13. Does the child leave an instruction half finished	often 0	sometimes ½	seldom or never 1
14. How does the child play the blow-organ, the Melodica etc.?	very badly 0	clumsily ½	fluently 1
15. Does the child make writing errors, even to the extent of having to rub out or cross out what he was written?	often 0	sometimes ½	seldom or never 1
16. Does the child move cautiously, not smoothly?	often 0	sometimes ½	seldom or never 1
17. Does the child like to draw in short lines or small parts instead of in big, sweeping lines?	often 0	sometimes ½	seldom or never 1
18. Does the child bump into other children?	often 0	sometimes ½	seldom or never 1
19. Does the child walk with his feet turned outwards?	markedly so 0	moderately ½	not at all 1
20. When the child has to crawl underneath something, does he do so clumsily, for example by not bending down far enough and thus bumping his head, or loosing his cap or hat (say a paper hat at a party)?	often 0	sometimes ½	seldom or never 1
21. Does the child walk with legs wide apart?	markedly so 0	moderately ½	not at all 1

22.	Does it ever happen that the child does not foresee what consequences his actions may have, e.g. when unscrewing something (so that the whole lot comes tumbling down), pushing something so far aside that there is not enough room left for something else, etc.?	often 0	sometimes $1/2$	seldom or never 1
23.	Does the child make mistakes in his drawings, so that he has to rub it out and do it again?	often 0	sometimes $1/2$	seldom or never 1
24.	Does the child have little accidents such as dropping things, bumping into things, knocking things over etc.?	often 0	sometimes $1/2$	seldom or never 1
25.	Does the child walk with his feet turned inwards?	markedly so 0	moderately $1/2$	not at all 1
26.	Are any of his movements angular (small jerks)?	most 0	some $1/2$	practically none 1
27.	Does the child spill his food when eating?	often 0	sometimes $1/2$	seldom or never 1
28.	(For girls) Can the child skip with a rope, play at fives, catch a ball? (For boys) Can the child wip a spinning top, play football, using his best foot straight away, catch a ball, throw a ball?	practically unable to 0	clumsily $1/2$	very capably 1
29.	Does the child forget where he puts things (mislays things)?	often 0	sometimes $1/2$	seldom or never 1
30.	Does the child stick out his tummy?	very much 0	fairly noticeably $1/2$	normal 1
31.	Is the child's speech rhythmic?	very unrythmic 0	rather forced $1/2$	fairly good 1
32.	To an order which demands quite a lot of movements, does the child execute it very slowly? (as it were well-thought out)?	often 0	sometimes $1/2$	seldom or never 1
33.	Is the child's walk straggling, unrhythmic and somewhat clumsy or stiff?	very strongly 0	appreciably $1/2$	not at all 1
34.	Does the child hold his ballpoint or pencil clumsily when writing and/or drawing?	often 0	sometimes $1/2$	seldom or never 1
35.	Does the child walk with his knees together? (knock-kneed)	markedly so 0	moderately $1/2$	normal 1

36. Does the child loose sense of time? Does he also have difficulty in understanding what for example a quarter past two means?
often 0   sometimes $1/2$ seldom or never 1

37. Does the child alternate right and left hands, for example by writing with one hand, and drawing and eating with the other?
often 0   sometimes $1/2$ seldom or never 1

38. Does the child enjoy routine jobs, such as simply copying writing or figures, jigsawing from a picture and so on, actions which require little thinking and planning?
markedly so 0   moderately $1/2$ seldom or never 1

39. Does the child use word-groups, sentences?
seldom or never 0   sometimes $1/2$ often 1

40. Does the child require support when going up and down the stairs?
often 0   sometimes $1/2$ seldom or never 1

Sum: .... + ... = ...

Figure 35

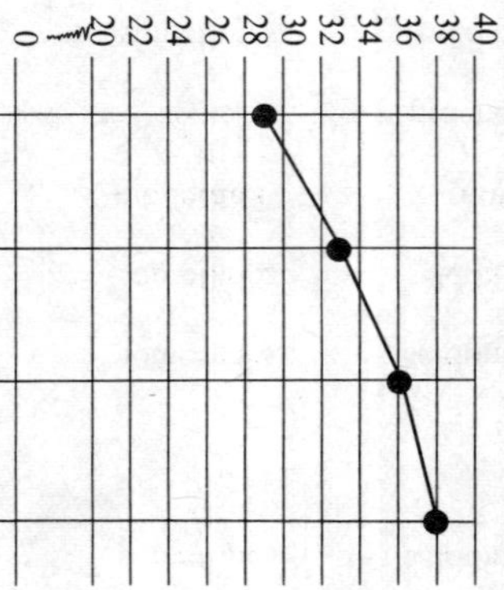

Age	7;6 N. 24	8;6 N. 24	9;6 N. 27	10;6 N. 23
Average	29	33	36	38
Stand. dev.	5	7	7	9

132

Table 42.
Standardisation of the Inventory for eupraxic behaviour of prelingually profoundly deaf children 7 to 10 years of age (max. 40)

Age	Number of children involved	Average scores
7;6	24	29 ± 5
8;6	24	33 ± 7
ceiling: 9;6	27	36 ± 7
10;6	23	38 ± 9

Table 43.

Tests	Bergès and Lézine	Rhythm Test	Inventory
Bergès and Lézine		.72	.68
Rhythm Test			.62
Inventory			

All correlations were significant p < 0.001.

All 95 children were observed by me, the class teacher and the speech teacher, to get some indication of their speech ability. This resulted into the following χ^2 distributions of the data of the last observation, which appeared to be highly significant (Table 44).

Similar distributions, also significant, have been found for the Bergès and Lézine and the rhythm-test for deaf preschool children.

"Oral fluency"
Ad (13) "Speaking as many words as possible within 2 minutes". Test of oral fluency.

Table 44.

Speech	Eupraxia inventory for preschool children			
	< 26 p.c. rank	26 - 75 p.c. rank	> 75 p.c. rank	Total:
Good progress	1	17	14	32
Moderate progress	2	33	7	42
Retarded progress	15	5	1	21
Total:	18	55	22	95

χ^2 68.938 df. 4 p < 0.001

In hearing children Tinker et al. (1940) found a correlation of 0.83 between an oral fluency in the form of quickly finding many associations in words, and their vocabulary. This was confirmed by Gerwitz (1948 a, b). In 51 deaf children we found a correlation of 0.47 (p < 0.01) between our oral fluency-test (taken at the ages of between 7;0 and 10;10) and the reading scores of the same children two years later ("Metropolitan Paragraph Reading Test", taken between the ages of 9;6 and 13;3). In 11 children between 8;7 and 10;5 years old a correlation of 0.69 (p < 0.05) was found between their oral fluency and their verbal IQ according to the Wechsler WISC, whereas the correlation with the performance IQ was only 0.28 (not significant). In 22 children aged between 10;6 and 12;5 these correlations were 0.64 (p < 0.01) and 0.43 (p < 0.05) respectively. We conclude that this oral fluency test is quite a reliable measure of the verbal development of deaf children, and also that it concerns the content of the words, not the speech technique.

"Lipreading-hearing-imitating-test"
Ad (14) "Lipreading with sound perception and repeating".
In five classes the validity of this test was examined, with the help of a comparison in pairs of the children by their own teacher: "Which child speaks and lipreads better?". We found the following significant correlations between the result of the test and the teacher's opinion: group of 7-year olds: 0.83, group of 9-year olds 0.74, group of 10-year olds 0.77, group of 11-year olds 0.82 and group of 13-year olds 0.88. The significance-level is always < 0.01. This test seems therefore to be a valid

measure of lipreading-sound-perception-speech, taken as one whole. The "split-half"-technique was applied to the scores of 35 children by comparing the even and odd items: this resulted in a rank-correlation of 0.87 (p < 0.01).

b. Observations concerning factors I and II

Factor I:

(a) The problem of the strong memory for simultaneously presented visual data

The polarity of factor I showed that the children who reacted quickly motorily were weaker in the memory tests for simultaneously presented data, and conversely, that the children who reacted less quickly motorily, achieved better results in these memory tests. Were both categories of children responsible to the same extent for this contrast? Hiskey (1966) gives for his tests "memory for colours" and "memory for pictures" standard scores, which can be expressed in "IQ-notations". Thus we could compare the total "Hiskey-IQ" per child, to be found in our files, with the standard scores per test. We divided each group into two halves: one half comprised those children who scored lower in the total results of the tests for "fluent fine motor function", the other half were those who scored higher
We found the following (Table 45).

In the memory test for simultaneously presented pictures it appears, especially among the three youngest groups, that the eupraxically more fluent children often appear somewhat weaker than their IQ would indicate. The dyspraxic children appear stronger. Thus these latter groups of children seem to be more responsible for the contrast. These findings are similar to those mentioned above, page 75. Can one *explain* this connection between dyspraxia and this particularly strong memory?

We suggest an answer via the so-called short-term memory and via the "set" or the child's attitude or anticipation-pattern. In the "changing class" of our observation centre, we observed deaf children aged about 2 years. Even at that young age one child seems to be more dexterous than the other. At that age we cannot yet administer tests for intransitive movements, but the difference is clear enough in the *transitive* movements such as dressing oneself and building blocks, at least at that age, because the difference seems to disappear when the children are about 4 years old. For example, both types of children are playing with a ring-tower; they have to put rings of different sizes and colours onto a pin. The dexterous children soon finish it, – it seems as if the temporal

135

Table 45.
"Fluent fine motor function"

Grouping of the children	Number of children and average age	Average IQ according to Hiskey's test	Memory for simultaneously presented coloured rods in "IQ-notations"	Difference with IQ	Memory for simultaneously presented pictures in "IQ-notations"	Difference with IQ
Children who scored lower in fluent fine motor function	Group I N = 10, 7;5	109 ± 16	111 ± 17	+ 2	129 ± 21	+ 20
	Group II N = 9, 8;3	108 ± 9	119 ± 17	+ 11	133 ± 20	+ 25
	Group III N = 12, 9;3	103 ± 13	106 ± 9	+ 6	108 ± 17	+ 5
	Group IV N = 11, 10;5	109 ± 12	108 ± 19	− 1	116 ± 20	+ 7
Children who scored higher in fluent fine motor function	Group I N = 10, 7;4	108 ± 13	106 ± 16	− 2	106 ± 19	− 2
	Group II N = 9, 8;6	109 ± 7	104 ± 17	− 5	114 ± 19	+ 5
	Group III N = 11, 9;5	106 ± 14	104 ± 11	− 2	106 ± 12	0
	Group IV N = 11, 10;6	99 ± 18	106 ± 17	+ 7	96 ± 12	− 3

succession of the actions also appears to them more or less as one entity. The less dexterous children take a longer time. They do see a result, which they achieve through trial and error, but their memories have difficulty in surveying the order of the series of actions, because it takes them such a long time and also because their actions are less directed. May we assume that these children, provided they have normal intelligence and memory, develop a kind of "set" by which they orientate themselves to the present, the simultaneous datum? Hearing children too can be clumsy, but in them the difficulty in surveying can be compensated by speech, certainly in the long run, via the "echoic memory". This is not the case with congenitally deaf children.

(We found some normally hearing children, however, who, suffering from a very weak speech memory, reacted like deaf children, in this respect.)

(b) Typical reactions to auditory training
The function of sound perception has not been investigated in this research. It will be treated elsewhere (in press). It must be mentioned here, however, that deaf children scoring lower in fluent fine motor function score significantly lower too in our auditory multiple choice spondee-test, sometimes notwithstanding considerable residual hearing.

The two poles of factor I make one think of the contrast between dancing movements (in acoustic or sound perceptive space) and executions of movements in optical space, in which the latter function more or less simultaneously as reference-frameworks. It must be remarked that, by definition, hearing is a stronger successive process than seeing.

(c) Dysphasia in the sense of dyspraxia of speech
An analysis of the speech-errors which the dyspraxic children made in the "lipreading with perception and repeating" test (14), produces the following picture:
- an impeded differentation of the mouth-positions, e.g. the difference between /a/ and /o/ and such like (e.g. lamanade instead of lemonade);
- impeded control of the order of phonemes (monolade);
- perseverations (e.g. lolomade);
- substitutions (e.g. letolade);
- omissions (e.g. lolade);
- additions (e.g. lemonolade);
- uncoordinated voice and articulatory movement, e.g. cap may become gab or cab;
- unpredictability of speech-errors;
- a quickly forgotten speech-pattern (e.g. the word lemonade is re-

peated correctly once, but when it has to be repeated from memory it may become lemode, lomade, loom, lade...);
- difficulty in imitating longer words, i.e. the greater the dyspraxia, the more difficult the imitation will be for the child, e.g. "residential", "triangular" (this also applies to complex idioms and sentences, with as a consequence dysgrammaticism);
- impeded lipreading, inclusive of impeded listening.

In short: difficulties with the *"speech-plan"*. Together with the phenomenon of an impeded memory for successive data (see factor I) all this makes one think of the description of patients with motor aphasia by Prick and Calon (1950, 1967) and the disorder in the "gnosis of body-activity-relation", disorder in the control of the "body scheme", which lies at the root of this, according to Prick (1959).

(d) Integration of the written and the spoken forms of words
The fact that the test "speaking as many words as possible within 2 minutes" (13) is found among the memory tests for simultaneously presented data, probably points to the following. When one looks for a connection between spoken word and simultaneously presented data, the first thing one's attention is drawn to is the written form of the words. Test (13) being among the memory tests mentioned can indicate that, verbally, a certain integration took place between the written word and the spoken word. The eupraxic children did less well in this test than the dyspraxic ones. We may conclude from this that the written word is important to all deaf children as a support to their verbal ability, and also that the "clumsy speakers" need not lag behind in language because of their dyspraxia. Has, in the case of the eupraxic children, too little attention been paid to a good integration of the written and spoken word? This might mean an important pointer in their didactics.

(e) Eusymbolia as content-symbol-integration
There must be an integration between the words and their meanings. A smooth integrative function in this respect can be called: eusymbolia (van Uden, 1980). Test (13) is concerned with the content of the words. This is in contrast with the other tests on learning to speak (14) and (15), which try to approach the more technical side of speech: e.g. the test-words of the lipreading-test are by no means known to all the children. The smooth integration between the written and spoken forms of the words (= the function of eulexia-dyslexia-alexia) seems to be related to eusymbolia-dyssymbolia-asymbolia, on the basis of sensori-motor integrative functions. This aspect is the topic of another research of ours, still in progress: eusymbolia and eulexia are based upon the fundamental function of sensori-motor integration (van Uden, 1977).

138

Factor II:

(a) Activity and motivation

This factor II seems to indicate that difficulties in remembering successively presented visual data go hand in hand with passivity in the child. This becomes especially clear in the group of 8-years olds. The only test in which these children scored on average lower than the 7-year olds is no. (6): "simultaneous digit-symbol association".

The 7-year olds scored on average 32.3 ± 7.5, and the 8-year olds 27.4 ± 5.2 (t = 2.134 p < 0.05). In all of the publications we know (e.g. Getz, 1953; K. Murphy, 1957; Clarke and Leslie, 1971) deaf children on average scored significantly lower in this test than hearing children; their scores in this test were the lowest of all of the WISC performance sub-tests.

It should be noted, however, that slowness in attack and execution of tests is characteristic of deaf children. If the experimenter is aware of this, he will take particular care to motivate the child to work quickly. When one motivates the deaf children correctly, their score is normal. For example, the average standard-score of the 83 children in this test is 11 and 12, respectivly, in no way different from the other tests. The scores of this group of 8-year olds, however, were exceptional. Does this show a passive, possibly insufficiently motivated attitude?

(b) Activity and memory function

Whereas the tests for successively presented data do not load on factor I, they do affect factor II, in contrast with two tests for remembering simultaneously presented visual data. The importance of this factor, however, decreases with age, which seems to mean that the difference between simultaneous and successive data decreases as regards the achievements of the children, apart from the drawing tests which do not load on this factor. We worked out the differences between the scores in simultaneous presentation of the pictures in test (3) and in presenting them successively in test (4), in which retardation of the successive element as opposed to the simultaneous one was considered as a lower score and the levelling with or the exceeding of this successive element as

NB. *Correlations with hearing-loss and intelligence (Table 46).*
Product-moment correlations have been computed between the scores of the 15 selected tests and
  performance IQ – WISC;
  hearing-loss in dB (Fletcher index, ISO)
and the understanding of spondee words by a multiple choice from 25.
The subjects were all of the children of the research of the syndrome of dyspraxia, 7-10 years of age, N = 83.

opposed to the simultaneous one as a higher score. In the 83 children there appeared to be a correlation of 0.64 with the calender-age, and of 0.76 with "fine rhythm of the mouth", the test which according to factor II demanded most activity from the child. Both correlations were significant (p < 0.001). The difference between the simultaneous and the successive elements consequently decreases with age and this is somehow linked with the increasing development of activity in the child.

Table 46.

15 selected tests	Correlations with performance IQ	Correlations with hearing-loss in dB	Correlations with correct identifications of spondee words
1. "Memory for colours"	+ .53**	+ .22*	+ .09
2. "Paper folding'"	+ .16	+ .08	+ .52**
3. "Visual Attention Span"	+ .54**	+ .17	+ .01
4. "Memory successive pictures"	+ .38**	+ .14	+ .45**
5. "Digit Span"	+ .31**	+ .04	+ .53**
6. "Digit Symbol"	+ .68**	+ .19	− .02
7. "Benton Drawing"	+ .64**	+ .18	− .06
8. "Benton Identification"	+ .68**	+ .30**	− .13
9. "Knox' Cube"	+ .39**	+ .15	+ .36**
10. "Bergès and Lézines"	+ .05	+ .12	+ .52**
11. "Finger movements	− .03	+ .10	+ .46**
12. "Rhythm"	− .10	+ .01	+ .60**
13. "Oral fluency"	+ .37**	+ .31**	+ .23*

14. "Lipreading"	− .07	− .07	+ .72**
15. "Memory for speech"	− .05	− .02	+ .56**
Identification of spondees by sound perception	− .17	− .56**	
Hearing-loss in dB.	+ .29**		− .56**
Performal intelligence		+ .29**	− .17

** = significance p < 0.01
 * = significance p < 0.05

8. CONCLUSION

The problem of this research can be answered as follows:

There is a "syndrome of dyspraxia" to be found in many deaf children.
In the 83 children examined, the 15 tests could mainly be divided into two groups: on the one hand those for eupraxia, on the other, those for memory for simultaneously presented visual data. At the same time this revealed two types of children: *eupraxic types* with a somewhat weaker memory for the simultaneously presented data mentioned, and *dyspraxic types* whose memory for these data was extremely strong. We call this phenomenon:

The syndrome of dyspraxia in deaf children.

Speech appeared to be supported by two poles: among the tests for eupraxia were those for the more formal articulatory aspect of speech; among the memory tests mentioned were those for speech content. This difference increased with age, to the extent that the dyspraxic children were using the strong side of their memory. These "dyspraxic deaf children", especially in the beginning, were the "clumsy speakers", but they gradually conquered their handicap: their language acquisition was not behind that of the eupraxic ones.

There are "active" and "passive" deaf children, but this difference is gradually conquered.
The tests could be grouped in yet another way, i.e. those which demand-

141

ed activity from the child and two tests in which the child could saturate simultaneously presented visual data. Here too, two types of children revealed themselves, the active ones and the passive ones. Learning to speak seemed to demand a special activity from the deaf child, as all the tests which are connected with speech were in the active pole. This difference in type of children, however, decreased with age.

At the same time it appeared that the difference between achievements in simultaneously presented visual data and those in successively presented data gradually disappeared.

The relatively unaffected phenomenon: speech.
Of all the memory-tests the ones for spoken words appeared relatively unaffected, at all ages and also in children who showed a weaker memory, which phenomenon can probably be explained by a greater routine in same: the children were completely oral and used speech all the time.

Consequences for practical teaching.
In children who learn to speak fluently, the integration of this speech with the written word and the memory of this written word should not be neglected. On the contrary both should be stimulated, because the ready availability of words seems to be connected with that memory. This applies even more strongly to children who do not learn to speak so fluently. For them the written word should be promoted too, because, they, more than anyone else, have to learn to make the written word support their speech. It appears that they are able to do this, because they had their words, plus the spoken forms, more readily available than the fluent speakers.

Ways should be found to conquer a too passive visual behaviour, to which some children are inclined. This behaviour hampers a good development of speech, which seems to require a strongly active attitude by deaf children. One has to try to achieve a good routine in speech, which is only possible when the child is continuously stimulated in a speaking environment.

Summary
Can we find any factors which influence speech-training favourably or unfavourably? Because speech appeared to progress especially at the ages of between 7 and 10 years, four groups of children were composed, aged respectively 7 (numbering 20), 8 (18), 9 (23) and 10 (20). They were prelingually deaf children without additional handicaps, who had a performance IQ of more than 90. The four groups did not differ significantly from each other as regards their IQ, average learning ability and hearing-loss. From a battery of 32 tests with which the children were investigated, 15 were chosen which according to experience were more

directly related to learning to speak. Four of these tests concerned the "supple use of the mouth when speaking", three, the "fluent fine motor function", three, "the memory for successively presented visual data" and five concerned "the memory for simultaneously presented visual data". Regarding the last, one should think of the written image as an important support for speech-training.

From the results of the tests spread over the four groups, product-moment correlation matrices were composed which were subjected to an INDSCAL-3-factors' analysis. The three factors found were: factor I, a polar factor – "eupraxia versus simultaneous visual cognition"; – factor II, again a polar factor, "active-passive", and factor III, a negative factor, "forget-factor". As far as the last is concerned, which was about equally important in all age-groups, children who scored highly in this appeared to have failed in non-routine memory tasks. Memory-tasks which incorporated speech appeared to be relatively less affected, probably because of the greater routine. According to factor I there appeared to be two kinds of children: those with fluent fine motor function who scored a little less in memory tests for simultaneously presented visual data, and others who were less fluent motorily, but reacted extremely well in exactly those memory tests mentioned. The contrast became more pronounced the older the children were; this indicates that the dyspraxic children started to use their memory-reserves increasingly better. According to factor II there also appeared to be two types of children: those who did well if they could absorb simultaneously presented visual data passively, but less well if they had to be active, including executing memory-tasks for successively presented visual data; and children who were more or less the inverse. This contrast, however, diminished, the older the children were, in favour of a more active behaviour by all the children. Where speech-training is concerned, an analysis of the imitation of speech by dyspraxic children indicated typical speech-errors, connected with less correct coordination of the "speech-plan" and memory for speech. Concerning the content of speech every child somehow seemed to rely heavily on his memory for simultaneously presented visual data, which must be the written image of the words.

VII. Does seeing oneself speak benefit lipreading?

A help especially for dyspraxic deaf children?

Introduction

Lipreading is an important component in learning to speak. If it can be furthered, one may reasonably expect better speech through an improved *visual* control.

When studying the relation between lipreading and speech we should realize that we do not see ourselves speak, unless at some time, in front of a mirror. One can *listen* to one's own speech, check one's *articulation*, e.g. "What is the position of my tongue when speaking /oo/? How do I position my lips?"

Seeing ourselves speak in front of a mirror gives a kind of "reafferent perception" (Von Holst and Mittelstaedt, 1950). One could also call this a visual feedback, a controlling loop (Frank, 1964; Voorhoeve et al., 1971) between speech and lipreading.

In most lipreading methods one exclusively practises in reading from someone *else's* lips. Visual proprio-*per*ception is omitted. Yet, it is suggested (Gesell, 1940) that this proprio-perception forms as it were a bridge to the correct perception of others. Other methods often use the mirror. The mirror has been seen as a useful instrument in learning to lipread and speak by deaf children for a long time (van Helmont, 1697; Amman, 1692), and is also used by those who became deaf at a later age (see Kooi, 1924; Jeffers and Barley, 1971). To rectify speech errors, Burkland (1967) used a videorecorder both in closed-circuit TV (i.e. a direct connection between camera and monitor without videorecording) and in recording. The videorecorder offers more opportunities than a mirror: one can enlarge pictures of the mouth, one can give side-views, make videorecordings and show them afterwards, etc. Larr (1959) had done the same when teaching people who had become deaf, to lipread; he showed them their "speaking face", just the mouth, face and upper part of the body, a front view and side-view, etc.

When the video set is used in closed-circuit TV, there is synchronous "reafferention" of one's own speech. However, when one first records this speech and then shows it to the patient, one gets successive self-perception, "proprio-*perception*".

All this concerns the making aware of aspects in speech and lipreading. The visual proprio-perception of own speech may also unconsciously influence improvement of lipreading. A comparative study into the effect on lipreading of this (conscious) seeing of one's own speech in comparison with exclusively seeing other people's speech has not yet been done.*

1. PROBLEM

Our problem reads as follows: Can lipreading be furthered without various aspects being made explicitly conscious? Is lipreading furthered by a synchronous or by a successive visual perception of own speech? Does the latter method have advantages over an exclusive learning by reading from someone else's lips? The advantages of feedback can be: the training-time may be shorter; the gain in lipreading is greater; there is more transfer from practised words to non-practised ones, and/or more transfer from lipreading from known persons to lipreading from unknown persons.

2. SUBJECTS, ALL OF THE INSTITUTE FOR THE DEAF, SINT MICHIELSGESTEL

Forty-eight prelingually profoundly deaf boys were chosen who could read and speak. They were aged between 8 and 14 years, divided into 4 groups of 12, which groups were equal as regards the following criteria:
(1) Hearing-loss, in dB, ISO-standard, Fletcher-index.
(2) Performance IQ, Snijders-Oomen non-verbal Intelligence Test (data supplied by Mrs. Drs. M. Guffens-Stoopman, who had examined these children at least twice from infancy).
(3) Chronological age.
(4) Results of an oral fluency test (speaking as many words as possible within 2 minutes), as a measure of speech orientation.

---

* The video-equipment needed for the experiment to be described below has been generously placed at the author's disposal by "Philips Gloeilampenfabrieken N.V." at Eindhoven.

(5) The results of Brus's "One-minute-test" (1963): the child has to read quickly and correctly increasingly more difficult words for 1 minute. Maximum score is 100. This is a measure both of reading and of speech.
(6) Results of Benton's test: memory for designs.
(7) Results of Knox' Cube test: reproducing patterns of movements.
(8) Results of "Lipreading with soundperception and repeating" test.

The tests (4) up to and including (8) are aimed at having comparable groups as regards speech, lipreading, memory for simultaneously and successively presented visual data, see Tables 47, 48, 49 and 50.

Subjected to Kruskal-Wallis's standard (Edwards, 1963) there appear to be no significant differences between the groups.

3. PRESENTED MATERIAL: HOMORGANIC WORDS

The material consisted of lists I and II, each of 32 nonsense-words (according to Dutch).
(1) Nonsense-words were used. If normal words had been used, the knowing or not-knowing of the words would have played a role in recognizing and repeating them.
(2) The words were composed of the vowel /a/ (as in bah), combined with so-called homorganic or homophenous consonants, which have a common articulation-point. Groups of 4 words were made for the exercises:

List I (32 words)
1. lat – lan – nal – tal
2. dans – nans – sans – tans
3. natta – tatta – tanda – tanna
4. tan – nat – tat – nan
5. mamp – mampa – mabba – mappa
6. kang– kank – kach – kaj (j =y as in yet)
7. gach – gak – gaj – gank
8. hak – haj – hach – hang

List II (32 words)
1. damma – tamma – madda – matta
2. tast – nant – nast – tant
3. nansa – tansa – dansa – nasta
4. stat – stan – stant – dant
5. jak – jang – jach – jaj
6. chakka – kakka – kacha – kanka

Table 47.
Data on the 4 groups of children A, B, C and D, taking part in the test on the effect of 4 different methods of lipreading-training.

DATA ON THE SUBJECTS:

Group A.

Name	Hearing-loss on the best ear, dB	Performance IQ	Age	Oral Fluency	Brus max. 100	Benton max. 10	Knox max. 15	Lipreading max. 100	Pretest max. 64
C.D.	105	112	8;7	49	48	6	11	77	9
C.R.	105	108	11;8	48	62	3	13	85	12
A.H.	95	91	9;8	32	56	6	11	61	5
H.S.	110	92	11;5	34	49	5	14	58	4
B.S.	105	96	11;0	30	50	4	6	62	5
H.F.	105	100	11;0	29	11	6	11	37	3
B.H.	115	90	9;10	37	36	6	10	55	2
P.J.	110	95	9;8	26	35	5	12	78	8
J.L.	95	112	11;2	55	54	9	13	74	1
L.C.	110	117	13;6	46	76	8	13	81	6
K.T.	95	112	11;10	57	63	7	12	91	0
K.E.	110	94	14;3	24	49	7	10	80	6
Averages	105.00 ± 6.45	101.58 ± 9.47	11;0 ± 2;0	38.91 ± 10.90	49.08 ± 15.75	6.00 ± 1.58	11.33 ± 2.01	70.00 ± 14.58	5.08 ± 3.30

Tabel 48.
Group B.

Name	Hearing-loss on the best ear, dB	Performance IQ	Age	Oral Fluency	Brus max. 100	Benton max. 10	Knox max. 15	Lipreading max. 100	Pretest max. 64
P.J.	110	86	10;3	22	40	2	8	41	2
H.H.	100	89	10;2	22	25	6	10	39	2
J.S.	115	100	10;8	21	20	6	12	53	6
F.K.	95	104	11;4	15	37	5	12	67	7
K.G.	110	110	11;3	19	34	10	10	32	6
R.M.	95	100	11;2	33	39	7	10	38	3
R.B.	>125	100	11;2	43	50	7	9	58	5
H.O.	115	95	10;5	47	55	5	9	62	5
F.K.	105	104	12;1	56	64	8	11	63	2
J.W.	>125	90	10;4	54	67	8	10	85	18
W.S.	110	106	11;10	62	60	8	12	76	10
E.M.	105	117	12;7	62	64	7	10	91	5
Averages	109.00 ± 9.53	100.80 ± 7.32	11;0 ± 0;6	38.00 ± 17.19	46.25 ± 15.29	5.75 ± 2.10	10.25 ± 1.23	58.75 ± 18.29	5.91 ± 4.29

Table 49.
Group C.

Name	Hearing-loss on the best ear, dB	Performance IQ	Age	Oral Fluency	Brus max. 100	Benton max. 10	Knox max. 15	Lipreading max. 100	Pretest max. 64
P.R.	110	102	10;7	25	38	4	8	55	6
P.P.	110	108	9;0	26	51	7	9	69	7
J.W.	90	104	8;9	43	55	5	11	60	6
H.S.	100	122	8;5	32	52	5	11	78	2
L.J.	105	90	10;2	33	37	4	10	57	5
D.O.	95	94	10;3	36	40	8	11	56	8
M.H.	105	106	9;3	31	36	5	11	51	3
L.G.	105	95	11;4	32	69	7	9	62	4
A.K.	105	105	10;4	60	59	7	14	81	4
D.M.	115	104	11;5	56	49	8	9	62	4
J.V.	115	123	12;2	79	65	9	13	82	4
P.O.	90	92	11;8	55	66	6	10	84	10
Averages	104.58 ± 9.81	103.75 ± 10.12	11;1 ± 1;0	42.33 ± 15.91	51.41 ± 11.32	6.25 ± 1.58	10.41 ± 1.35	66.41 ± 11.36	5.16 ± 2.22

Table 50.
Group D.

Name	Hearing-loss on the best ear, dB	Performance IQ	Age	Oral Fluency	Brus max. 100	Benton max. 10	Knox max. 15	Lipreading max. 100	Pretest max. 64
K.P.	110	109	9;0	25	22	7	10	73	6
K.O.	95	116	8;5	31	52	6	11	54	8
D.K.	120	105	9;2	12	42	7	13	72	10
H.K.	110	108	9;0	35	43	6	11	89	19
T.R.	110	90	9;4	48	32	4	10	55	10
P.H.	90	88	11;1	39	33	5	10	72	8
E.P.	120	120	12;6	48	56	8	10	83	6
S.S.	110	114	14;0	49	58	9	11	89	6
B.B.	105	116	12;8	76	55	8	13	88	9
W.K.	90	114	14;8	46	31	8	13	79	7
E.K.	115	104	13;9	53	51	5	13	77	7
H.R.	105	98	13;4	63	60	5	11	69	5
Averages	106.25 ± 10.63	106.83 ± 9.98	11;0 ± 2;6	44.41 ± 17.17	44.58 ± 11.81	6.50 ± 1.50	11.33 ± 1.24	75.00 ± 11.34	8.41 ± 3.54

7. kanga – kanja – kaja – jaja
8. happa – hamma – hampa – hapma

The homorganic consonants connected with the same vowel are extremely difficult to distinguish in lipreading. This, however, can be practised. Non-homorganic nonsense-words would probably be too easy so that a difference in training-method, as formulated in the problem, would not show a significantly different effect.

4. PROCEDURE

a. Survey
Each group was treated as follows:
   First a pre-test was done in order to see how many nonsense-words were recognized. This was followed by a training period, and finally a re-test in order to measure a possible progress in lipreading.

b. The test-tape for pre- and re-test
A person unknown to the children spoke the 2 x 32 nonsense-words in random order (Table 51). These 64 testwords were preceded by four "trial words": mam, pam, map and pap, for instructive purposes.

A video sound-recording was made in the following way. The speaker was standing in front of the videorecorder's camera. His face and his neck were taken "en face". According to research by Larr (1959), this gives the highest intelligibility for lipreading, when using a "closed circuit television" monitor. The speaker looked into the lens of the camera so that he was looking at the child when the film was shown. He spoke the nonsense-words in an even tempo with no additional movements. After each word he paused for 10 seconds and the camera was blacked out. These 10 second pauses gave the child the opportunity to react when taking the test, which reactions were registered by two observers. This videotape will hereunder be called the "test-tape".

c. Test-procedure
The pre- and re-test were taken in exactly the same way, as shown in Figure 36.

The child was sitting in front of the videorecorder monitor; the size of the screen was 30 x 35 cm. The brightness and clearness of the picture were kept constant, as well as the light in the quiet room (artificial light from fluorescent tubes). The distance between the child's eyes and the picture was about 1 to 1.50 m (the best distance for lipreading, O'Neill, 1961).

Table 51.

Homophenous words.
N.B. The figures I and II do not concern the pre- or re-test, but the "transfer": certain children were only trained in the words marked I, others only in the words marked II. In both the pre- and re-test they were tested on all the words in order to see whether a transfer of training had taken place.

Random order of 64 homophenous words, recorded on a video-tape ("test-tape"), for the Pre-test and the Re-test.

Name of the child: ....Age: .....Form: .....Group A, B, C or D.
Name of the observer: ....*Testwords:*   *Notes:*

Introductory words:		*Notes:*	*Testwords:*			*Notes:*
a. mam		....	30. mabba	I		....
b. map		....	31. kakka	II		....
c. pap		....	32. nal	I		....
d. pam		....	33. hamma	II		....
Testwords:			34. yaya	II		....
1. happa	II	....	35. gay	I		....
2. tal	I	....	36. matta	II		....
3. stat	II	....	37. dans	I		....
4. gank	I	....	38. nat	I		....
5. hang	I	....	39. nansa	II		....
6. tanna	II	....	40. yang	II		....
7. tast	II	....	41. gak	I		....
8. kang	I	....	42. kagga	II		....
9. dansa	II	....	43. tant	II		....
10. kay	I	....	44. kanya	II		....
11. kag	II	....	45. hak	I		....
12. kaya	II	....	46. sans	I		....
13. nans	I	....	47. nant	II		....
14. stan	II	....	48. tanda	I		....
15. nan	I	....	49. mampa	I		....
16. tat	I	....	50. mamp	I		....
17. tatta	I	....	51. yag	II		....
18. gakka	II	....	52. lan	I		....
19. kanka	II	....	53. stant	II		....
20. lat	I	....	54. nasta	I		....
21. yaya	II	....	55. dant	II		....
22. kank	I	....	56. madda	II		....
23. kamma	II	....	57. hampa	II		....
24. hag	I	....	58. kanga	II		....
25. hay	I	....	59. tamma	II		....
26. natta	I	....	60. hapma	II		....
27. mappa	I	....	61. tans	I		....
28. nast	II	....	62. tansa	II		....
29. tan	I	....	63. yak	II		....
			64. gag	I		....

153

Figure 36.

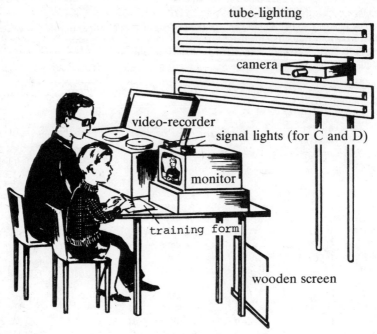

Arrangement of a training session.

Two observers, taking notes, who were familiar to him (a co-worker and the author), were sitting diagonally behind him, at a distance of about 50 cm, so that he could not see their faces. The child did not use a hearing-aid: we were only concerned with pure lipreading.

We first tried it out on other boys to see whether the arrangement was satisfactory. Because the two observers could not lipread very well, the loudspeaker of the videorecorder had to remain connected. The volume, however, was reduced to 20-30 dB, which could not possibly be perceived by children with a hearingloss of over 90 dB. This loudspeaker was standing on another table so that the children could not feel any vibrations.

Before the test was carried out, the experimenter used the videorecorder only in the closed-circuit arrangement, for an initial instruction. He spoke a few words: Institute (the child repeated it), Sint-Michielsgestel (ditto), post-office (ditto), ball (ditto), without the sound being switched on.

154

NB. Most children were surprised that the sound was not switched on. Some did not want to take off their hearing-aids, when they understood what was happening.

However, after some explanation ("You will learn from it") the situation was accepted by all the children.

Then the camera was switched off, the recorder and test-tape were switched on and shown on the monitor.

Both observers had a copy of the form (see Table 51) in front of them. On it were all the words in the same order in which they appeared on the tape. The form was not shown to the child. Both observers wrote down what the child said after each word, sometimes two words when the child spoke two words because he was uncertain or in order to correct himself. The latter word was regarded as the real response.

On the whole the children's behaviour was quiet and attentive. Some of them were somewhat tensed up and felt a bit frustrated at first. This, however, improved when we showed them at the trial word stage that everything they said was per se "right".

d. Scoring
Scoring was done in the following way. Each observer noted down independently what he thought the child said. Afterwards the notes were compared. Only the "items" which were noted down as being *correct* by *both* observers were regarded as being correct.

e. Training
The children were trained in one of the two lists only, thus in 32 words; 6 children of each group were trained in list I and the remaining 6 in list II. Nevertheless, in the pre- and re-test all of the 64 words were shown, so that we could see whether there was any progress in lipreading as far as the 32 non-trained words were concerned: which indicates a transfer of training.

Each child was individually trained by the experimenter, in 4 sessions of about 15 minutes, according to 17 forms (first the instruction-form a. + 2 times 8 training-forms, each for 4 homorganic words).

The training-method was identical for all the children, with the exception of one aspect per group (A, B, C and D).

Initially we used the trial series for each child as an instruction, as follows:
The experimenter and the child were sitting together in front of the monitor. The experimenter put the first form in front of the child:

Articulation-check:	mam map pap pam	
Training-series:	mam mam mam mam mam	
	map map map map map	
	pap pap pap pap pap	one "block"
	pam pam pam pam pam	
Lipreading-check:	map mam pam pap pap mam map pam	

At this point the video apparatus had not yet been switched on. The experimenter started by *checking the articulation,* i.e. he checked whether the child could pronounce correctly the four words in question. (In fact this appeared sometimes to cause a difficulty with the following three words only: *kanja, kanga* and *hapma.* These problems were soon overcome.) The experimenter pointed to the first written word *mam,* asked the child to look at him and said *mam.* The child imitated this. Then the same with *map,* and *pap* and *pam.* After that he asked the child to read the four words unaided. If this was done without difficulty, the training proper started.

This training was done in the following way:

The video apparatus was switched on. The experimenter pointed to the first word of the "block": *mam,* and asked the child, who was facing the monitor, to pronounce it.

This occurred as follows. The experimenter moved his right hand first up and then down and thus he and the child spoke at the same time, synchronously, *mam.* They did this five times at a regular tempo of about one word every 2 seconds.

The same was done with *map,* and *pap* and *pam.*

When the whole block was finished, *lipreading* was *checked,* i.e. whether the child could lipread the words from the experimenter. The experimenter took the form away from the child and asked him to look at him. He pronounced the four words, twice, in random order as is given on the form: map...mam...pam...pap...pap...mam...map...pam. As appropriate the experimenter showed either his approval or disapproval. All the mistakes were written down by him. If the child made no more than one mistake then he was considered able to lipread these words. If there was more than one mistake, they started on the second *trial* on this form, if necessary on the third trial and in extreme cases on the fourth. Here the exercise stopped, even if the child was still making more than one mistake.

After this trial-series the first form of the real training was started, namely part 1.

"lat – lan – nal – tal" (I)
or "damma – tamma – madda – matta" (II).
When the first part had been treated in the way described above, they proceeded to the second part, etc. Examples: see Table 52.

The exercise comprised four sessions of 15 minutes each. In these four sessions the child was presented with all his words (32) twice, in the first session, parts 1, 2, 3 and 4, in the second session, parts 5, 6, 7 and 8. In the third session, parts 1, 2, 3 and 4 were treated again and in the fourth session, parts 5, 6, 7 and 8.

In order to avoid a possible recency- or starting-effect, the order of the parts was reversed for every other child: for example child G.O. was presented with the usual order, parts 1-2-3-4 and 5-6-7-8, but child F.R. with the reverse order 4-3-2-1 and 8-7-6-5.

The whole shows an "embracing" arrangement, see page 162.

Four different training-methods
In each of the four groups of children one change was applied in the training-method. We will explain this on the basis of the trial series described above.

Group A.
The child sees himself speaking on the monitor right at the start. Synchronous self-perception.

The videorecorder is used in a closed-circuit TV arrangement. The camera is focussed onto the child, so that he can see his face and neck "en face" on the monitor. The experimenter lifts his hand and when he lowers it, the child says *mam*, synchronously with the movement of the hand. This was done five times. Further the procedure is as described above.

Group B.
The child sees the experimenter speaking on the monitor, in synchronism with his own speech.
Synchronous perception of another person.
Everything is exactly as under A, except that the camera is aimed at the experimenter and that both speak synchronously when the hand moves. The child does not see himself speaking, he only sees the experimenter.

Group C.
The child speaks and sees himself speaking afterwards; i.e. he reads from his own lips.
Successive self-perception.

157

Table 52.

Three examples of the training-forms: The trial-series for the instruction, list I part 3, and list II part 5.

Form for lipreading-training (trial series)

Name of the child: .... Age: ..... Form: ..... Group: .....
Date of training: ....

Trial words to explain the instruction.

Articulation-control: mam   map   pap   pam   Remarks, if any:

a. Tape-numbers: ..... to .....
   mam   mam   mam   mam   mam
   map   map   map   map   map
   pap   pap   pap   pap   pap
   pam   pam   pam   pam   pam

Lipreading-control:
map .... mam .... pam .... pap ..../pap .... mam .... map .... pam ....

b. Tape-numbers: ..... to .....
   mam   mam   mam   mam   mam
   map   map   map   map   map
   pap   pap   pap   pap   pap
   pam   pam   pam   pam   pam

Lipreading-control:
map .... mam .... pam .... pap ..../mam .... pap .... map .... pam ....

c. Tape-numbers: ..... to .....
   mam   mam   mam   mam   mam
   map   map   map   map   map
   pap   pap   pap   pap   pap
   pam   pam   pam   pam   pam

Lipreading-control:
map .... mam .... pam .... pap ..../pap .... mam .... map .... pam ....

d. Tape-numbers: ..... to .....
   mam   mam   mam   mam   mam
   map   map   map   map   map
   pap   pap   pap   pap   pap
   pam   pam   pam   pam   pam

Lipreading-control:
map .... mam .... pam .... pap ..../mam .... pap .... map .... pam ....

158

Form for lipreading-training.

Name of the child: .... Age: ..... Form: ..... Group: .....
Date of training: ....

List I part 3.

Articulation-control: natta tatta tanda tanna   Remarks, if any:

a. Tape-numbers: ..... to .....

natta	natta	natta	natta	natta
tatta	tatta	tatta	tatta	tatta
tanda	tanda	tanda	tanda	tanda
tanna	tanna	tanna	tanna	tanna

Lipreading-control:
tatta ... tanda ... tanna ... natta ... / tatta ... tanna ... tanda ... natta ...

b. Tape-numbers: ..... to .....

natta	natta	natta	natta	natta
tatta	tatta	tatta	tatta	tatta
tanda	tanda	tanda	tanda	tanda
tanna	tanna	tanna	tanna	tanna

Lipreading-control:
tatta ... tanda ... tanna ... natta ... / tanna ... tatta ... tanda ... natta ...

c. Tape-numbers: ..... to .....

natta	natta	natta	natta	natta
tatta	tatta	tatta	tatta	tatta
tanda	tanda	tanda	tanda	tanda
tanna	tanna	tanna	tanna	tanna

Lipreading-control:
tatta ... tanda ... tanna ... natta ... / tatta ... tanna ... tanda ... natta ...

d. Tape-numbers: ..... to .....

natta	natta	natta	natta	natta
tatta	tatta	tatta	tatta	tatta
tanda	tanda	tanda	tanda	tanda
tanna	tanna	tanna	tanna	tanna

Lipreading-control:
tatta ... tanda ... tanna ... natta ... / tanna ... tatta ... tanda ... natta ...

Form for lipreading-training.

Name of the child: ....   Age: ..... Form: ..... Group: .....
Date of training: ....

List II part 5.

Articulation-control: yak   yang   yag   yay   Remarks, if any:

a. Tape-numbers: .....to .....

yak	yak	yak	yak	yak
yang	yang	yang	yang	yang
yag	yag	yag	yag	yag
yay	yay	yay	yay	yay

Lipreading-control:
yak ....yag ....yang ....yay ..../yay ....yag ....yang ....yak ....

b. Tape-numbers: .....to .....

yak	yak	yak	yak	yak
yang	yang	yang	yang	yang
yag	yag	yag	yag	yag
yay	yay	yay	yay	yay

Lipreading-control:
yak ....yag ....yang ....yay ..../yag ....yay ....yang ....yak ....

c. Tape-numbers: ......to .....

yak	yak	yak	yak	yak
yang	yang	yang	yang	yang
yag	yag	yag	yag	yag
yay	yay	yay	yay	yay

Lipreading-control:
yak ....yag ....yang ....yay ..../yay ....yag ....yang ....yak ....

d. *Tape-numbers: .....to .....*

yak	*yak*	*yak*	*yak*	*yak*
yang	*yang*	*yang*	*yang*	*yang*
yag	*yag*	*yag*	*yag*	*yag*
yay	*yay*	*yay*	*yay*	*yay*

Lipreading-control:
yak ....yag ....yang ....yay ..../yag ....yay ....yang ....yak ....

In order to prevent the glass of the monitor functioning as a mirror or distracting the child's attention, a screen is placed between the child and the monitor. The camera is aimed at the child as in A. The child's speech is recorded on videotape. As soon as the whole "block" of 20 words has been worked through the experimenter rewinds the tape and takes the screen away, so that the film may be shown.

Above the monitor are two lights, a red light on the right and a white one on the left. The film is played back, the child reads from his own lips and repeats each word. If his response is correct, the experimenter signals with the white light, if it is not, he uses the red one. The number of mistakes are counted.

Group D.
The child and the experimenter speak synchronously. Afterwards the child sees only the experimenter speak, i.e. he lipreads from the experimenter. This is successive perception, first articulatory from himself, then visually from someone else.

The camera is now aimed at the experimenter. As in B he speaks synchronously with the child. Only the experimenter's speech is taped and shown to the child afterwards. The future procedure is the same as in group C.

5. RESULTS

The raw scores, consisting of the correctly repeated words of the test-tape, are given here in averages with their standard deviations, according to the "embracing" scheme shown in Tables 53 and 54.

The gain in the re-test. Analysis of variance
A variance-analysis on our data was carried out, with the help of the computer programme Varian/03 (Kwaaitaal and Roskam, 1968). Co-operator Van der Sanden arranged the results in the following survey:
"The following facets (factors) are included in the design:
Factor N: subject saw spoken image *immediately* versus *afterwards*
factor O: subject saw himself *versus* the experimenter
factor P: subject is trained in List I *versus* List II
factor Q: subject was presented with the words in the *usual order* versus *reverse order*
factor S: the *subjects* (N=48).
factor R: *pre-test* and *re-test*

N.B. Factor S is embraced by the factors N, O, P and Q.

Table 53.
Survey of the "embracing" test arrangement.

Pre-test: 48 children; lipreading 64 homorganic nonsense-words (list I and II, mixed) spoken by an unknown person (videotape).

	Group A (N 12) 1 see themselves speaking synchronously		Group B (N 12) see only the experimenter speaking synchronously		Group C (N 12) have to read from their own lips		Group D (N 12) have to lipread from the experimenter	
	Trained with list I (N 6)	Trained with list II (N 6)	Trained with list I (N 6)	Trained with list II (N 6)	Trained with list I (N 6)	Trained with list II (N 6)	Trained with list I (N 6)	Trained with list II (N 6)
Training 2	↓ (N3)	↑ (N3)	↓ (N3)	↑ (N3)	↓ (N3)	↑ (N3)	↓ (N3)	↑ (N3)
3	↑ (N3)	↑ (N3)	↑ (N3)	↑ (N3)	↑ (N3)	↑ (N3)	↑ (N3)	↑ (N3)

Re-test: the same 48 children; lipreading from the same videotape used for pre-test.

↑ : usual order of the parts 1-2-3-4 and 5-6-7-8.
↓ : reverse order: 4-3-2-1 and 8-7-6-5.

Table 54.

Pre-test

	List I	List II
Group A 5.08 ± 3.29	2.08 ± 1.78	3.00 ± 2.13
Group B 5.92 ± 4.48	2.92 ± 2.75	3.00 ± 2.21
Group C 5.17 ± 2.33	2.75 ± 1.81	2.42 ± 1.44
Group D 8.42 ± 3.70	4.75 ± 2.33	3.66 ± 2.18

Re-test

		Trained with I	Trained with II
Group A 11.0 ± 3.97	Gain 5.92 ± 3.26	9.17 ± 3.99	12.83 ± 3.66
		↑ 10.0 ± 5	↓ 14.33 ± 4.51
		↑ 8.33 ± 2.52	↓ 11.33 ± 2.52
Group B 8.58 ± 4.98	Gain 2.67 ± 1.77	7.83 ± 4.45	9.33 ± 5.78
		↓ 11.33 ± 3.21	↓ 9.00 ± 1.00
		↑ 4.33 ± 1.53	↑ 9.67 ± 9.07
Group C 12.0 ± 5.04	Gain 6.83 ± 5.57	11.0 ± 5.40	13.0 ± 4.69
		↑ 12.66 ± 5.69	↓ 12.0 ± 1.73
		↑ 9.33 ± 6.12	↑ 14.0 ± 7.00
Group D 10.92 ± 7.49	Gain 2.50 ± 4.21	10.33 ± 4.76	11.50 ± 8.85
		↓ 10.0 ± 3.46	↑ 16.33 ± 11.15
		↑ 10.66 ± 6.65	↑ 6.66 ± 1.15

The design was a multifactor experiment with repeated measurements, N, O, P and Q being between-subjects factors and R within-subject factor.

Because most of the effects appeared to be very non-significant (most of them even had an F ratio smaller than 1), we are giving part of a variance-analysis in Table 55, in which *only* the error-terms, against which was *tested*, all the main effects and the other effects having an F ratio greater than 1, are included. This will also provide a better survey."

Table 55.
(Incomplete) Variance-Analysis Table.

Variance source	df.	MS	F
1. Error between (subjects within groups)	32	9.68	
2. N	1	.84	.087
3. O	1	86.26	8.914**
4. P	1	1.76	.182
5. Q	1	17.51	1.809
6. Residue within (i.e. R Subj. within groups + N O P Q R)	33	7.85	
7. R	1	25.01	3.186*
8. O R	1	10.01	1.275
9. P R	1	11.34	1.445
10. N Q R	1	17.51	2.230
11. N O P R	1	17.51	2.230
12. N O Q R	1	8.76	1.116
13. N P Q R	1	10.01	1.275

** $p < .01$ (df: "degrees of freedom"; MS: "mean square")
* $p < .10$

(Conclusion of van der Sanden's report.)

Consequently we see that seeing oneself speak is the only factor which gives significant gain in this test, and that no other interaction was significant.

Further comparisons of the data
Application of the "difference-test" and the "t test for difference of two averages" (Edwards, 1963) teaches the following:

(a) A matrix of comparisons between the groups A, B, C and D according to the results of the pre-test (absolute scores) by means of the "t test for difference of two averages" are given in Table 56.

Table 56.

Group M	A 5.08 ± 3.29	B 5.92 ± 4.48	C 5.17 ± 2.33	D 8.42 ± 3.70
A 5.08 ± 3.29		t = 0.510 p = 0.615	t = 1.179 p = 0.671	t = 1.788 p = 0.087
B 5.92 ± 4.48	N.S.		t = 1.866 p = 0.075	t = 1.860 p = 0.076
C 5.17 ± 2.33	N.S.	N.S.		t = 1.845 p = 0.078
D 8.42 ± 3.70	N.S.	N.S.	N.S.	

As regards the absolute scores of the pre-test, the differences between the groups are not significant.

(b) All the groups show significant *gain* in the *re-test* compared with the pre-test (Table 57).

Table 57.

Group	Pre-test	Re-test	Difference	Difference-test	Significance
A	5.08 ± 3.29	11.0 ± 3.97	+ 5.92 ± 3.26	6.287	p = 0.00005
B	5.92 ± 4.48	8.58 ± 4.98	+ 2.67 ± 1.77	5.203	p = 0.0003
C	5.71 ± 2.33	12.0 ± 5.04	+ 6.83 ± 5.57	5.091	p = 0.00005
D	8.42 ± 3.70	10.92 ± 7.49	+ 2.50 ± 4.21	5.344	p = 0.0003

(c) Matrix of *comparisons* between the groups A, B, C and D according to the results of the *re-test* (absolute scores) by means of the "t test for difference of two averages" (Table 58).

Table 58.

Group M	11.0 A ± 3.97	8.58 B ± 4.98	12.00 C ± 5.04	10.92 D ± 7.49
A 11.0 ± 3.79		t = 1.313 p = 0.202	t = 1.5643 p = 0.132	t = 1.837 p = 0.08
B 8.58 ± 4.98	N.S.		t = 1.863 p = 0.076	t = 1.855 p = 0.077
C 12.00 ± 5.04	N.S.	N.S.		t = 1.854 p = 0.077
D 10.92 ± 7.49	N.S.	N.S.	N.S.	

As regards the absolute scores of the re-test, the differences between the groups are not significant.

(d) Matrix of *comparisons* between the groups A, B, C and D according to the *gains* by means of the "t test for difference of two averages" (Table 59).

As regards gain, the groups A and C score significantly higher than B and D. C scores somewhat higher than A, but this difference is not significant, nor is it for B with respect to D. This produces the following order:

C = A > B = D

The transfer of training per group
In the first place there is a certain transfer in so far that all the groups lipread better after the training-period, even from an unknown speaker.
   The most important transfer, however, concerns a gain in the words in which the children were *not* trained.

When we measure this transfer of training against the average gain which the children achieved in the *non-trained words,* we see the following (Table 60).

166

Table 59.

Group M	5.92 A ± 3.26	2.67 B ± 1.77	6.83 C ± 5.57	2.50 D ± 4.21
5.92 A ± 3.26		$t = 3.677$ $p = 0.001$	$t = 0.492$ $p = 0.627$	$t = 3.531$ $p = 0.002$
2.67 B ± 1.77	S.		$t = 2.979$ $p = 0.007$	$t = 1.776$ $p = 0.089$
6.83 C ± 5.57	N.S.	S.		$t = 2.805$ $p = 0.010$
2.50 D ± 4.21	S.	N.S.	S.	

Table 60.

Group	Average gain in non-trained words	Average gain in trained words	Difference-test	Significance
A	2.83 ± 2.95	3.08 ± 1.99	0.240	$p = 0.87$
B	0.33 ± 2.35	2.33 ± 2.10	2.174	$p = 0.04$
C	3.17 ± 3.16	3.67 ± 3.37	0.371	$p = 0.81$
D	0.50 ± 0.75	2.00 ± 3.76	1.340	$p = 0.18$

Groups B and D appear to obtain their significant gain in the re-test almost solely from the words in which they were trained.

The difference between the gain in practised words and that in non-practised words is significant in group B, in favour of the practised words.

In groups A and C the gain is practically the same, both for the words in which they were trained and for those in which they were not trained. This difference is not significant, so that we can speak of a *transfer of training.*

The number of trials necessary in training
In all the groups the number of trials decreased, as Table 61 shows (series 1, 2, 3 and 4):

Table 61.

Group	Number of trials M		Difference	Difference-test	Significance
	series 1 + 2	series 3 + 4			
A	20.25 ± 4.81	14.08 ± 2.81	− 6.17 ± 3.67	5.670	p = 0.0001
B	20.75 ± 6.02	16.50 ± 4.06	− 4.25 ± 4.49	3.275	p = 0.07
C	20.83 ± 4.36	13.00 ± 3.33	− 7.83 ± 4.11	6.605	p = 0.00004
D	15.58 ± 4.62	12.17 ± 3.99	− 3.41 ± 2.61	4.535	p = 0.0009

The number of trials necessary for the group A and C showed the greatest decrease; the difference is significant with respect to the groups B and D (t = 3.0592, p = 0.002). The greater decrease in group C with respect to group A is not significant (t = 0.935, p = 0.33).

We found the following product-moment-*correlations* between the degree of gain in the re-test and the decreases in the number of trials in the various groups:

Group A .53 not significant
Group B .47 not significant
Group D .41 not significant
Group C .56 p < 0.10.

6. ADDITIONAL TEST OF REACTION-TIME

It occurred to us that, when taking the re-test in the groups A and B, the A-children repeated the words fluently and at a regular tempo, whereas the B-children reacted irregularly and hesitantly, which often did not contribute towards the correctness of their reactions.

Problem: Do the tempo and the regularity with which the children repeat the spoken words have anything to do with learning to lipread?

Subjects: The children in groups C and D.

Procedure: When taking the pre- and re-tests the reaction-time was determined as follows:

As soon as a word had been spoken on the monitor (i.e. at the last speech-sound) the stopwatch was started and as soon as the child started to talk (at the first speech-sound) it was stopped. The stopwatch was accurate to 1/10 of a second. This space of time was noted down per item.

The average, with its standard-deviation, of the 64 reaction-times was worked out for each child. This standard-deviation is treated as a measure of the regularity of the reactions. After all when a child reacts to the spoken image on the monitor at a constant tempo, this means that the standard-deviation of his reaction-time is small, and vice versa.

Results:
(a) The regularity in the reaction-time.
The difference in reaction-speed between the pre- and re-test was negligible, see Table 62.

Table 62.

Group	Average reaction-time in seconds		Difference-test	Significance
	Pre-test	Re-test		
C	2.38 ± 0.97	2.15 ± 0.56	1.157	p = 0.272
D	2.61 ± 0.74	2.41 ± 0.66	2.742	p = 0.019

Although both groups show a slight acceleration in their reaction-times (0.23 and 0.20 seconds respectively) only group D's is significant ($p < 0.02$). There were two children in group C whose reactions deviated because they were slower than those of the rest, which caused the correlation comprised in the test to be too low.
The regularity of reaction is more important, see Table 63.

Table 63.

Group	Regularity of reaction in seconds		Difference-test	Significance
	Pre-test	Re-test		
C	0.68 ± 0.35	0.48 ± 0.24	2.506	p = 0.029
D	0.65 ± 0.40	0.61 ± 0.39	1.336	p = 0.21

When taking the pre-test, nearly all of the 24 children reacted rather irregularly, with standard deviations of more than half a second. This remained the same in group D. In group C, however, the regularity increased significantly up to a standard deviation of less than half a second.

(b) Relation to gain.
We worked out order-correlations between the degree of regularity in

169

reaction-time (standard deviations of the reaction-times) and the degree of gain achieved in the re-test, which gave the results shown in Table 64.

Table 64.

Group	Pre-test	Significance	Re-test	Significance
C	+ 0.15	p > 0.05	+ 0.60	p < 0.02 sign.
D	+ 0.29	p > 0.05	+ 0.34	p > 0.05 not sign.

Group C's regular reaction in the re-test is positively and significantly related to the degree of gain.

7. DISCUSSION

(1) First a few remarks about the experiment as such.

(a) Not all the 64 words were completely (Dutch) *nonsense-words*, e.g. "lat", "dans", as we found out later. Cooperator Smulders, an expert in Dutch, found 15 meaningful words. For this reason, after the experiment, we investigated further to see of the difference between "meaningful" words and "nonsense" words had played a part in the children's reactions. The percentages of correct identifications in pre- and re-tests were worked out. This showed no significant difference in correct identifications:
 "meaningful" words N=15, M=15.34% ± 8.956
 "nonsense" words N=49, M=12.43% ± 11;76
 t=0.992 p=0.381.

(b) Were both the list I and II *equally difficult* for learning to lipread? The average scores of the two lists were compared with each other, see Table 65.

Table 65.

	Average number of correct reactions		Difference-test	Significance
	List I	List II		
Pre-test	2.43 ± 2.39	2.27 ± 2.26	0.186	p = 0.853
Re-test	5.70 ± 2.69	4.92 ± 3.47	1.656	p = 0.104

170

No significant difference in difficulty was found.

(c) The two observers for pre- and re-test:
The *variability in markings* of the two observers was investigated. Only those words which were put down as being correct reactions by both observers were regarded as correct. There were 805 reactions which were judged to be correct by both observers, and 21 about which their opinions differed (i.e. 2.54%). These 21 reactions were divided among the groups and tests as shown in Table 66.

Table 66.

	Pre-test	Re-test	
Group A	3	3	The variability in the observers' markings,
Group B	2	3	evenly divided among the groups,
Group C	4	2	does not seem to have influenced the result.
Group D	2	2	

(d) *Group D* scored the least gain of all the groups, but in the pre-test they scored significantly higher than the others. Had this group perhaps reached the ceiling of their abilities with these extremely difficult words? No, as in the re-test the absolute scores of groups A and C were higher than those of D. In principle D should have been able to achieve higher scores.

(e) The training was done only by *the experimenter* himself. Did this not involve a risk that he would involuntarily train certain groups more intensely than others? This is a real danger. Therefore the arrangement of the training-method was strictly formal, so that a possible personal influence did not contribute towards the various results. See p. 155.

(2) Progress in "lipreading"?
All the groups individually showed a significant progress in the lipreading of a series of nonsense-words. This was to be expected, because the situation had become more familiar to them in the re-test, and the material was more or less described. The latter facilitates a correct reaction by mere guessing. To what extent can the results be explained in this way? In other words, had the lipreading as such of these 64 words become more effective, or only the familiarity and/or guessing from material described?

Whether lipreading as such has indeed improved can be deduced on the one hand from improved identification of very small speech-con-

171

trasts, on the other hand from improved lipreading in everyday life. The first cannot be concluded from the results, the latter can hardly be expected after such a short training-period of only four sessions each lasting about 15 minutes.

Can more effective guesswork explain the progress? Probably not. Only half of the words were trained. The number of correct identifications of *non*-trained words had increased as well. What about familiarity? A greater familiarity with the lipreading-*situation*, which is an important factor in the development of lipreading (Jeffers and Barley 1971), seems indeed to be an acceptable explanation. This familiarity would particularly arise in children who had seen themselves speak (groups A and C). The lipreading-situation in our experiment was: lipreading nonsense-words, which were very difficult to discriminate, from an unknown speaker. The situation is certainly one of the most difficult possible. Although it is always risky to draw generalized conclusions from one single experiment with a limited number of subjects, one may nevertheless expect that analogic effects will occur in less difficult lipreading situations, e.g. one works with known words, word-groups and sentences. Further tests will have to show whether in addition refined perception of speech-contrasts may be an effect of this training-method.

(3) Seeing oneself speak and familiarity in *the lipreading-situation*.
How can seeing oneself speak have any influence on a greater familiarity in the lipreading-situation? We would describe "greater familiarity" as an absence of fear of failure, feeling at ease, abandonment. – The following four explanations seem feasible. One could say that the subjects who had seen themselves speak controlled the situation more consciously. However, no attempt was made in this experiment to make the aspects of lipreading conscious. Of group C one could say that reading one's own lips had an exceptionally motivating effect, and of group A that the "contiguity" (E. R. Guthrie, 1959, quoted by Foppa, 1966) of seeing and speaking was stronger than in group B, with probably a stronger association between the two. The two explanatory possibilities come together in one fourth: the course of development from proprio-ception with proprio-perception to perception of others. One can compare seeing oneself speak, in this case reading from one's own lips, and thus achieving better lipreading from others, with the development of a baby, who at first looks at his own hand movements which in time develops the ability to grasp objects (Gesell, 1940).

The effects of a conscious, systematic treatment will also have to be examined further, particularly as to whether this method will facilitate

NB. See Smits' experiment (1975).

172

learning to speak: e.g. whether certain speech-sounds ("optemes"), tempo, rhythm of speech and memory for speech are favourably influenced. The research by Smits (1975) showed these effects.

(4) The different number of presentations.
The number of presentations of the nonsense-words to the subjects was not the same in all the groups. Might this be an explanation of the differences between the groups?

In all the groups the words were presented in written form, the experimenter spoke them first, the children had to repeat them and afterwards had to lipread from the experimenter and speak the words. This meant five presentations. In groups A and B the repeated speech and seeing of the spoken word on the monitor were added factors (seven presentations). In groups C and D there was also the repeated speech, with lipreading of the spoken words afterwards on the monitor and repeating (eight presentations). On the basis of this one could expect groups C and D to give the best training effects, which was not the case. Obviously the frequency of the presentation did not play a part.

(5) Feedback processes?
This has to do with the automation of the relation between lipreading and speech. Van der Veldt (1928) and Montpellier (1933) found a relation between the regularity with which a motor task was performed, and its automation, i.e. its relatively independent and autonomous functioning: rhythmic movement causes automation, and automation, by speeding up and repeating a movement, causes rhythmicity. Van Galen (1974) found something similar as regards speech of hearing people in a speech reaction-time experiment. The regularity with which group C reacted to lipreading by speech, points in the direction of automation and their speech becoming autonomous, a kind of sensory-motor Gestalt-formation.

(6) Do these children *visualize their own speech?*
Vahle (1929) was already pleading for the use of a mirror when teaching deaf children to speak, in order to unify speech and lipreading, which would enhance the speed of the conversation. The results of our experiment seem to indicate that this unification is improved when deaf children are trained in seeing their own speech.

How can lipreading and speech be unified? After all one does not see oneself speaking under normal circumstances.

We can control many of our movements, not only via peripheral perception, but centrally via our imagination. Ballet dancers who train in front of mirrors "see" themselves dance when they perform (Hartong, 1948). In this case one could speak of "search images" (Lersch, 1966) or, in general, of "mental pictures". We could describe the ballet dancers' experience as follows: they control the dance form through optical mental pictures of their own dance movements. The same may be said of the "mental training" in sport (cf. Cratty, 1967).

Do the results of our experiment indicate that deaf children can develop mental pictures of their own speech, analogous to the behaviour in performing dances and in sport? We believe we have to confirm this. The children in the experiment who had seen themselves speak, achieved better lipreading from a speaker unknown to them, i.e. at a moment when they no longer saw themselves peripherally. They also achieved transfer of training for words in which they had not been trained. The children who had not seen themselves speak did not get quite as far. In all this, seeing oneself, although not peripherally, appeared to be a significant factor.

An influence of visual mental pictures seems to show itself even more clearly in group C. The children in this group who had not seen themselves speak synchronously had to read from their own lips afterwards. The visual form of their speech was somewhat disconnected from their actual speech. In the same group C the reaction-time from lipreading to repeating seemed to become more regular, which indicates a certain integration of visual and spoken speech forms, thus a unity of lipreading and speech at which Vahle (1929) aimed.

(7) The reaction of Group C.

The day before the re-test was taken the children in this group had had a party which lasted until after midnight. They, however, went to school at the usual time next day. Both observers did not know about this, and were surprised at the children's tired reactions and yawning. Nevertheless their results were extremely good, but the observers were convinced that they could have been even better. The results of this group were in all aspects better than those of the other three groups. They had the sharpest decrease of the number of trials in training, the highest absolute score in the re-test, most gain in comparison with the pre-test and most transfer. The connection between training and gain was most obvious with them too.

The children's motivation during training was exceptionally good. Lipreading from themselves was completely new to them, but their reactions to it were positive in spite of their surprise that they had so much difficulty in understanding themselves. This stimulated them to increasingly improve their speech, which indicates a more and more conscious selfcontrol.

Moreover this method forces as it were the children to look at themselves; we can only assume that the children in group A did the same. Though the higher scores were not significantly better than those of

174

group A, this method seems to have special advantages. Further experiments could shed light on this. (See Smits 1975.)

8. CONCLUSION

The lipreading situation on which this experiment was based entailed lipreading nonsense-words which were very difficult to lipread, from an unknown speaker. The conclusions from this experiment are *as follows*:

By training, lipreading can also be developed without making the various aspects of it conscious, at least on the basis of a greater familiarity with the lipreading situation.

In the above lipreading situation, lipreading is developed more by training in seeing one's own speech than in seeing other people's speech. The advantages are clearly shown in the following findings: less training was necessary; the results when lipreading from an unknown speaker were better; there was more transfer to nonsense-words which were not practised. A group of children who had been trained with the same material by reading their own lips reacted more regularly when repeating words uttered by unknown speakers than a group who had only been trained in lipreading from someone else. There appeared to be a positive connection between this regular reaction and the gain in lipreading from an unknown person.

A consequence for practical teaching (see Smits, 1975):
One may reasonably expect that when deaf children are trained in seeing their own speech, their lipreading will improve. This training can be done extremely well by means of a video-set, both in closed-circuit TV and in video recording. When the children manage to lipread from themselves in video recording, we can be sure that they do indeed examine their own speech. They spontaneously tried to articulate more clearly. One should start by practising with words which they can speak, commencing with series of contrasting words and thus progressing to series of homorganic words. One can practise with rhythmically spoken word-groups, increasing the tempo of speech and further with sentences which one continues to extend. This method is recommended especially for *dyspraxic* children, who have lipreading difficulty.

Smits (1975), guided by us, executed a learning experiment, using visual delayed feedback by video-recording as in group C, using known words, word-groups and sentences, on five profoundly deaf students of 15 years of age, who were suffering from dyspraxia of speech and had great difficulty in lipreading, although they had had special treatment from early childhood (individual speech-training, lipreading and auditory training). The "Lipreading-hearing-imitating-test", was used as

175

pre- and re-test. The training period comprised 3 months, 25 hours altogether. The results showed a dramatic, highly significant gain of 31% (pre-test being M = 42% ± 18, re-test M = 73% ± 12 p < 0.001).

NB. Purposely no control-group was used in this research, because it is almost impossible to control all variables involved. Such comparisons with control-groups often look more scientific than they really are. It seems to be sufficient to have shown that the method worked within an unexpectedly short time.

This method of training lipreading (generally speaking, the students like it) is in use now for all pupils who have problems in lipreading at the Institute for the Deaf, Sint-Michielsgestel. – The first main effect is an increased feeling of security, feeling of familiarity with the lipreading situation explained above. The second main effect is that the child tries to improve his speech.

Improvement was also noted in the following areas:
(1) the visual discrimination of "optemes" and of rhythm-patterns,
(2) the tempo of speech, and
(3) the memory for spoken sentences.

Summary

Does seeing one's own speech promote lipreading? This question links up with a noted development from proprio-*perception* to perception of others: when lipreading is developed as proprio-perception, will this then influence lipreading as perception of others? Here a proprio-perception without making the children expressly aware of the various aspects of same is meant. One can appeal to proprio-perception via a mirror or video-equipment. In our test the latter was used. Four comparable groups of 12 prelingually deaf children were formed. The procedure was as follows: doing a pre-test, a training-period and setting a re-test. Pre- and re-test were identical. One video tape was used: someone unknown to the children spoke 64 homorganic nonsense-words; the children had to lipread and repeat them; the scores consisted of the number of words correctly repeated. The children were only trained in half of the 64 words, in order to see whether there was a transfer of training with respect to the non-trained words. Each group was trained in a different way. Group A: the child spoke and saw himself speaking synchronously on the monitor. Group B: the child spoke and saw only the experimenter speaking synchronously on the monitor. Group C: the child spoke, and saw himself speaking only on "play back", i.e. had to lipread from himself. Group D: the child spoke and saw afterwards only the experimenter speaking, i.e. had to lipread from the experimenter. The results showed significant gain in all the groups, but significantly most of all with the children who had seen themselves speaking: the

176

groups A and C. These last groups also needed significantly less training; there was significantly more "transfer of training". With the C and D groups the reaction-times were also taken down with pre- and re-test. Group C appeared to react significantly more regularly than group D in the re-test. Group C appeared to react better than all the other groups, both in training and in the re-test in every respect, but the difference with group A was not significant. The progress in lipreading can probably be explained by a greater familiarity with the lipreading situation. It was particularly marked in the case of the children who had seen themselves speaking. The result is a confirmation of the following process of development: via proprio-perception to perception of others.

This effect has been confirmed by an experiment carried out by Smits (1975) and guided by the author. Profoundly deaf children, suffering from the "syndrome of dyspraxia" showed a significant average gain of 31% in lipreading scores, after they had been trained to lipread their own speech patterns from a monitor. – This method is applied now to all pupils who have difficulty in lipreading at the institute for the Deaf, Sint-Michielsgestel.

Literature

A

Alich, G. "Zur Erkennbarkeit von Sprachgestalten beim Ablesen vom Munde", Universität Bonn 1960.

Alcorn, K. "Speech developed through vibration", Volta Review 1938 (40), p. 633-638.

Alcorn, S. "Development of speech by the Tadoma-method", "Proceedings of the 32nd Convention of American Instructors of the Deaf (CAID)", Washington D.C., S. Government Printing Office, 1941.

Ammann, J. C. "Surdus loquens, dat is wiskonstige beschrijvinge op wat wijse men doofgeborene sal kunnen leeren spreken", Haarlem 1692.

Ammann, J. C. "Surdus loquens, of de Dove Sprekende", Amsterdam 1697.

Anon., "Symposium 'De Stem'", Acta Physiologica et Pharmacologica Neerlandica 1956, p. 40-97.

Arnold, Th. "A method of teaching the deaf and dumb speech, lipreading and language", London 1881.

Aronson, E and Rosenbloom S., "Space perception in early infancy: perception within a common auditory-visual space", Science 1971 (172), p. 1161-1163.

B

Balen, C. van, "De verstaanbaarheid van excerpten uit opgelezen tekst en conversatie in het Nederlands: invloed van spreeksnelheid en duur van het excerpt", Amsterdam 1974.

Baker, H. J. and Leland B. "Detroit test of learning aptitude", University of Detroit 1959.

Bakker, J. "Stilleestest, bestemd voor het vierde leerjaar van de basisschool", Nijmegen 1969.

Barczi, G. "Hörerwecken und Hörerziehen", Salzburg 1936.

Bayley, N. "Mental growth during the first three years", New York 1935, 1969.

Bayne, Sh. "Vibro-tactile thresholds in pure tone audiometry", Unpubl. thesis Manchester University 1968.

Bean, C. "An unusual opportunity to investigate the psychology of language", The pedagogical Seminary and Journal of Genetic Psychology, XL 1932, p. 199-213.

Beaver, A. P. "The imitation of social contacts by pre-school children", Child Developm. Monographs no. 7, Teacher's College, Columbia University, New York 1932.

Becking, A. "Perception of airborn sound in the thorax of deaf children", Proceedings of the international course in paedo-audiology, Groningen 1953, p. 68-71.

Beertema, A. Koetsenruyter P., Postema P. and De Saint Aulaire R., "Spreekmotoriek en doofheid", Logopedie en Foniatrie 52, 1980, p. 146-160.

Bell, A. G. "Upon a method of teaching language to a very young congenitally deaf child", Washington D.C. 1884.

Bellugi, U. and Siple P. "Remembering with and without words", Problèmes actuelles de psycholinguistique, Colloque C.N.R.S., Paris 1971.

Benson, D. F. "Aphasia, alexia and agraphia", Churchill Livingstone, New York, Edinburgh and London 1979.

Benton, A. L. "Der Benton Test" (1953) Deutsche Bearbeitung von O. Spreen, Bern 1968.

Berger, K. W. "Speechreading principles and methods", National Educational Press, Baltimore, Maryland 1972.

Bergès, J. and Lézine S. J. "The imitation of gestures. A technique for studying the body scheme and praxis of children 3 to 6 (and 6 to 10) years of age", Paris 1963, London 1965.

Berkhout, P. R. "Spreekonderwijs aan dove kinderen", Amsterdam 1968.

Bieri, E. "Die Erscheinungsformen der Sprache und ihre Auswertung im Taubstummen und Schwerhörigen Unterricht", Schw. Ztschr. für Heilpädagogik 1944, p. 15-29. Groningen 1950, p. 53-61.

Birch, H. J. and Belmont, L. "Auditory visual integration in brain-damaged and normal children", Developmental Medicine and Child Neurology, 1965, p. 135-144.

Birdwhistell, R. L. "Kinesics and communication" in "Exploration in communication", Edm. Carpenter and M. Lc. Luhan eds. Boston 1960.

Birdwhistell, R. L. "The kinesic level in the investigation of the emotions" in Knapp P. H. ed. "Expressions of the emotions of man", New York 1963.

Birdwhistell, R. L. "Kinesics and context. Essays on body motion communication", Un. of Pennsylvania Press, Philadelphia 1970.

Biscaro, B. "L'aspetto fonetico del linguaggio nel sordo", Effatha 1970 (63), p. 123-128.

Bishop, M. E. Ringel R. L. and House A. S., "Orosensory perception in the deaf", Volta Review 1972, p. 289-298.

Bitter, G. B. and Mears, E. G. "Facilitating the integration of hearing impaired children into regular Public School Classes", Volta Bureau, Washington D.C. 1973.

Black, J. W. "Communication by voice", Naval Research Reviews 1965, p. 7-14.

Blank, M. and Bridger, W. "Conceptual cross-modal transfer in deaf and hearing children", Child Development 1966, p. 29-38.

Blevins, B. "The myth of 'Total Communication'", Am. Org. for the Ed. of the Hearing Impaired 1972, p. 2-6.

Bok, S. T. "Cybernetica. Hoe sturen wij ons leven, ons werk en onze machines?", Utrecht 1958, 1962.

Boothroyd, A. and Cawkwell S. "Vibrotactile thresholds in pure tone audiometry" Acta Oto-Laryngologica (Stockholm) 1970, p. 381-387.

Both, F. J. "Op school niet mee kunnen komen... en dan?", Swets and Zeitlinger B.V., Lisse 1982.

Brauckman, K. "Das Sprache-absehen vom Munde", Ztschr. f. Hals- Nasen- und Ohrenheilkunde 1923 (6), p. 155-160.

Brankel, O. e.a., "Vergleichende phoniatrische, Röntgenkymographische und ventilato-

180

rische Untersuchungen an hörenden und gehörlosen Versuchspersonen während der Ruhe und während des Sprechens", Phonetica 1965 (13), p. 162-182.

Breuer, H. and Weuffen, M. "Gut vorbereitet auf das Lesen- und Schreibenlernen", Deutscher Verlag der Wissenschaften, Berlin 1975.

Breuer, H. and Weuffen, M. "Untersuchung zum sprachlichen und verbosensomotorischen Niveau agrammatisch sprechender Vorschulkinder", Folia Phoniatrica 1977 (29), p. 177-190.

Brieland, D. M. "A comparative study of the speech of blind and sighted children", Speech Monographs XVII (no. 1 1950), p. 99-103.

Brill, R. G. "Administrative and professional developments in the education of the deaf", Washington D.C. 1973.

Broesterhuizen, M. Dijk, J. van and IJsseldijk, F. "Psychological and educational diagnosis and assessment", in Mulholland A. (ed), Washington D.C. 1980.

Brookshire, R. H. "A token test battery for testing auditory comprehension in brain-injured adults", Brain and Language 1978 (6), p. 149-157.

Broomfield, A. M. "Guidance to parents of deaf children, a perspective", British J. of Disorders of Communication 1967, p. 112-123.

Brown, J. W. "Aphasia, apraxia and agnosia, clinical and theoretical aspects", Springfield Ill. 1972.

Brown, R. and Bellugi, U. "Three processes in the child's acquisition of syntax", Harvard educ. Review 1964, p. 131-151.

Brown, R., Cazden, C. B. and Bellugi, U. "The child's grammar from I to III", in Ferguson and Slobin eds. 1973, p. 295-332.

Bruininks, R. H. "Bruininks-Oseretsky-Test of motor proficiency", American Guidance Service, Minnesota 1978.

Brus, B. Th. "Eén minuut-test", Nijmegen 1963.

Bryant, N. B. and Kass, C. E. "Leadership training institute in learning disabilities: Final Report Vol. 1 and 2, Tucson Arizona", University of Arizona 1972.

Bühler, K. "Sprachtheorie", Jena 1934.

Burkland, M. "Use of television to study articulatory problems", Journal of Speech and Hearing Disorders 1967, p. 80-81.

Buytendijk, F. J. J. "Het spel van mens en dier", Amsterdam 1932.

C

Caccamise, F. Blasdell R. and Meath-Lang B., "Hearing-impaired persons' simultaneous reception of information under live and two visual-motion media conditions", Working paper National Technical Institute for the Deaf 1976, abstract in Stuckless (ed). 1978, p. 15.

Callaway, E. "Brain electrical potentials and individual psychological differences", Grune and Stratton, New York 1975.

Calon, P. J. A. "Over de persoonlijkheidsontwikkeling bij kinderen met aangeboren of vroeg verworven doofheid", Nijmegen 1950.

Calvert D. R. and Silverman S. R., "Speech and deafness", Alexander Graham Bell Association, Washington D.C. 1975.

Campbell, H. W. "Phoneme recognition by ear and by eye", Kath. Universiteit Nijmegen, Psychologisch Laboratorium 1974.

Carr, J. "An investigation of the spontaneous speech sounds of five-year-old deaf-born children", Journal of Speech and Hearing Disorders 1953, p. 22-29.

181

Carr, M. J. "Communication behavior of three and four year old deaf children", Columbia University, New York 1971.

Carrol, J. D. and Chang, J. J. "Analysis of individual differences in multidimensional scaling via an N-way generalisation of 'Eckart-Young' decomposition", Psychometrika 1970 (35), p. 283-319.

Cazden, C. B. "Environmental assistance to the child's acquisition of grammar", Harvard University 1965.

Charrow, V. R. and Fletcher, J. D. "English as the second language of deaf students", Technical Report nr. 208 July 20 1973, Psychology and Education Series, Institute for mathematical studies in the social sciences, Stanford University, Stanford California.

Chen, H. P. and Irwin, O. C. "Infant speech vowel and consonant types", Journal of Speech Disorders 1946 (11), p. 27-29.

Clarke School for the Deaf "Clarke-School Studies", Northampton, Mass. 1970.

Clarke School for the Deaf "Curriculum series: Reading, speech, auditory training, word study, language, media", Northampton, Mass. 1972-1973.

Clarke, B. R. and Leslie, P. T. "Visual motor skills and reading ability of deaf children", Percept. Motor Skills 1971 (33), p. 263-268.

Cobb S., "Borderland of Psychiatry", Cambridge, Harvard University Press, 1948.

Connor, L. E. (ed), "Speech for the deaf child. Knowledge and use", Washington D. C. 1971.

Connor, L. E. Personal communication. 1972.

Conrad, R. "The deaf school child", Harper and Row, London 1979.

Cornett, R. O. "Cued Speech", American Annals of the Deaf, 1967, p. 3-13.

Cratty, B. J. "Movement behavior and motor learning", Philadelphia 1964.

Cratty, B. J. "Active learning", Englewood Cliffs N.J. 1967, 1971.

Cruickshank, W. M. (ed.), "Psychology of exceptional children", London 1956.

D

Dabout, Th. et Roinsol, J. "Automobile commandé par la voix", Revue Générale de l'Enseign. des Déf. aud. 1971, p. 167-168.

Dale, J. H. van en Kruyskamp, C. "Groot Woordenboek der Nederlandse Taal", Den Haag 1961.

Dale, D. M. C. "Deaf children at home and at school", London 1967, 2nd 1968.

Das, J. P. Kirby, J. and Jarman, R. F. "Simultaneous and successive synthesis: an alternative model for cognitive abilities", Psychological Bulletin 1975 (82), p. 87-103.

Das, J. P. Kirby, J. and Jarman, R. F. "The relationship between learning disability and simultaneous-successive processing", Journal of Learning Disabilities 1978 (11), p. 16-23.

Davis, H. and Silverman, S. R. (eds.), "Hearing and deafness", New York 1970.

Davitz, J. R. "The communication of emotional meaning", New York 1964.

Decroly, O. and Degang, J. "Contribution à la pédagogie de la lecture et de l'écriture", Archives de psychologie, Brussels 1907.

Deininger, M. "Das Problem der Früherziehung bei den Taubstummen", Eos, Vierteljahrschrift für die Erkenntnis und Behandlung jugendlicher Abnormen, Heft 5/6 Verl. Ferd. Berger in Horn, N.Österreich 1931.

Deleau, M. "Imitation des gestes et réprésentation graphique du corps chez les enfants sourds", Monographies Françaises de Psychologie (Red. P. Oléron), Education

Centre National de la Recherche Scientifique, Paris 1978.

DeRenzi, E. and Vignolo, L. A. "The Token-Test: a sensitive test to detect receptive disturbances in aphasics", Brain 1962 (85), p. 665-678.

Dewey,G. "Relative frequency of English speech sounds", Cambridge, U.S.A. 1923.

DiCarlo, L. M. "The effect of hearing one's own voice among children with impaired hearing", in Ewing A. W. G. (ed.) 1960, p. 37/1-14.

DiCarlo, L. M. "Some relationships between frequency discrimination and speech reception performance," J. aud. Res. 1962, p. 37-49.

DiCarlo, L. M., "Much ado about the obvious", Volta Review 1966, p. 269-273.

DiCarlo, L. M. and Brown, J. W. "The effectiveness of binaural hearing for adults with hearing impairments", J. aud. Res. 1960, p. 35-76.

Dijk, J. P. M. van, "Rubella handicapped children. The effects of bilateral cataract and/or hearing impairment on behaviour and learning", Swets & Zeitlinger B.V., Lisse 1982.

Dimond, S. J. "Neuropsychology. A testbook of systems and psychological functions of the human brain", Butterworths, London 1980.

Dongen, Br. A. van, "Tussen Aa en P. Fonetiek en articulatiecursus", Sint Michielsgestel 1957, 2nd 1962, Nijmegen 1970.

Downs, M. P. "Identification and training of the deaf child, birth to one year", Volta Review 1968, p. 154-158.

Driel, Zr. Theresia van, "Handleiding voor de beginnende doofstommenonderwijzer", St.-Michielsgestel 1934.

E

Edwards, A. L. "Statistical methods for the behavioral sciences", New York 1963.

Edwards, E. R. "A comparative study of form perception, kinesthetic and spatial orientation abilities in articulatory defective and normal speaking children", Purdue University 1970.

Eggermont, J. "De klankfrequentie in het hedendaags gesproken Nederlands", De Nieuwe Taalgids 1956 (49), p. 221-223.

Eggermont, J. "Taalverwerving bij een groep dove kinderen", Groningen 1964.

Elkind, D. (ed.) "National research conference on day programs for hearing impaired children", Proceedings, Al. Grah. Bell Ass., Washington D.C. 1968.

Elstner, W. and Karlstad, H. "Dysphasie im Kindesalter. Terminologie, Aetiologie, Rehabilitation, Integration" (German, English and French text), Universitetsforlaget Oslo - Bergen - Tromsö 1978.

Erber, N. P. "Speech envelope cues as an acoustic aid to lipreading for profoundly deaf children", Journal of the Acoustical Society of America 1972 (51), p. 1224-1227.

Erber, N. P. "Auditory, visual and auditory visual recognition of consonants by children with normal and impaired hearing", Journal of Speech and Hearing Research 1972 (15), p. 413-422.

Ertel, S. und Drost, R. "Expressive Lautsymbolik", Ztschr. exper. und angewandte Psychologie 1965 (12), p. 557-565.

Ewing, A. W. G. "Aphasia in children", London 1930, New York 1968.

Ewing, A. W. G. (ed.) "Educational guidance and the deaf child", Manchester 1957.

Ewing, A. W. G. (ed.) "The modern educational treatment of deafness", Manchester 1960.

Ewing, A. W. G. and Ewing, E. C. "Teaching deaf children to talk", Manchester 1964.
Ewing, A. W. G. and Ewing, E. C. "Hearing aids, lipreading and clear speech", Manchester 1967.
Ewing, A. W. G. and Ewing, E. C. "Hearing impaired children under five", Manchester 1971.
Ewing, A. W. G. and Ewing, I. "The handicap of deafness", London 1938.
Ewing, A. W. G. and Ewing,I. "Opportunity and the deaf child", Manchester 1951.
Ewing, A. W. G. and Stanton, D. A. G. "A study of children with defective hearing", The Teacher of the Deaf 1942, p. 127-134, 1943, p. 3-8, 26-30, 56-59.
Ewing, I. R. "The ascertainment of deafness in children under five years of age and their response to home-training", International Congress on the Care of the Deaf-mute, Groningen 1950, p. 101-111.
Ewing, I. R. and Ewing, A. W. G. "Deafness in infancy and early childhood", The Journal of Lar. and Ot., London 1943, p. 203-226.
Ewing, I. R. and Ewing, A. W. G. "Opportunity and the deaf child", London 1947, "New opportunities", London 1958.
Ewing, I. R. and Ewing, A. W. G. "Speech and the deaf child", Manchester 1954.
Ex, J. "Communicatie van gezicht tot gezicht", Nijmegen 1969.

F

Fairbanks, G. "Systematic research in experimental phonetics: a theory of the speech-mechanism as a servo-system", Journal of Speech and Hearing Disorders, 1954, p. 133-139.
Farnsworth, P. "The social psychology of music", New York 1958.
Ferguson, C. A. and Slobin, D. J. (eds.) "Studies of child language development" New York 1973.
Fisher, C. G. "Confusion among visually perceived consonants", Journal of Speech and Hearing Research 1968 (11), p. 796-804.
Flores d'Arcais, G. B. and Levelt, W. J. M. (eds.) "Advances in psycholinguistics", London 1970.
Foppa, K. "Lernen, Gedächtnis, Verhalten", Berlin 1966.
Fort, B. "Spontaneous vocalisations of two years old deaf children as related to the degree of hearing-loss and other factors", University of Kansas, Department of Education, 1955.
Forchhammer, G. "Absehen und Mundhandsystem", Blätter für Taubstummen Bildung, 1923 (36), p. 281-308, – in "Taubstummenpädagogische Abhandlungen", Leipzig 1930, p. 71-79.
Fraisse, P. "Rhythmes auditifs et rhythmes visuels", Année psychologique 1948 (49), p. 21-42.
Fraisse, P. "Les structures rhythmiques", Louvain 1956.
Fraisse, P. "Psychologie du rhythme", Presses Universitaires de France, Paris 1974.
Frank, H. "Lehrmaschinen in kybernetischer und pädagogischer Sicht", Stuttgart 1964.
Frisina, D. R. "Speechreading", Proceedings Intern. Congress on the Education of the Deaf, Washington D.C. 1963.
Fry, D. B. "Duration and intensity as physical correlates of linguistic stress", Journal of the Acoustical Society of America 1955, p. 765-768.
Fry, D. B. "The development of the phonological system in the normal and the deaf child", in Smith and Miller, G. A. "The genesis of language", New York 1966, p. 187-206.

Fry, D. B. "The physics of speech", Cambridge University Press, New York 1979.
Fucci, D. a.o. "Interaction between auditory and oral sensory feedback in speech regulation", Perceptual Motor Skills 45 (1), 1977, p. 123-129.
Furth, H. "Thinking without language", New York 1966.
Furth, H. "Deafness and learning, a psychological approach", Belmont California 1973.
Furth, H. and Youniss, J. "Thinking in deaf adolescents: language and formal operations", J. Comm. Dis. 1969, p. 195-202.

G

Galen, G. P. van "Ambient versus focal information processing and single-channelness", Kath. Universiteit Nijmegen, Psychol. Lab. 1974.
Gammon, S. A. Smith, P. Daniloff, R. and Kim, R. "Articulation and stress juncture production under oral anesthetisation and masking", J. of Speech and Hearing Research 1971, p. 271-282.
Gardner, A. R. and Gardner, B. T. "Teaching sign language to a chimpanzee", Science 1969, p. 664-672.
Garnett, C. B. "The exchange of letters between Samuel Heinicke and Abbé Ch. M. de l'Epée", Washington D.C. 1968.
Gates, R. "The reception of verbal information by deaf students through a television medium - a comparison of speech reading. Manual communication of speech reading", Proceedings of the Convention of American Instructors of the Deaf, Little Rock, Arkansas 1971, p. 513-522.
Gault, R. "On the identification of certain vowels and consonantal elements in words by their tactual qualities and by their visual qualities as seen by the lipreader", J. of abn. and soc. Psych. 1927, p. 29-41.
Gault, R. "Hearing by touch", The Laryngoscope 1927, p. 184-189.
Gebbard, J. W. and Mowbray, G. H. "On discriminating the rate of visual flicker and auditory flutter", Am. Journal of Psychology 1959 (72), p. 521-529.
Gerstmann, J. "Fingeragnosie und isolierte Agraphie. Ein neues Syndrom", Zeitschrift für die gesammte Neurologie und Psychiatrie 1927 (108), p. 152-177.
Gerwitz, J. L. "Studies in word-fluency. I. Its relation to vocabulary and mental age in young children, II. Its relation to eleven items of child behavior", J. Genet. Psychol. 1948 (72), p. 165-184.
Gesell, A. "The first five years of life", London 1940.
Getz, S. "Environment and the deaf child", Springfield Ill. 1953.
Ginneken, J. van "De roman van een kleuter", 's-Hertogenbosch 1922.
Gloyer, J. "Vergleich der leib-seelischen Entwicklung des gehörlosen Kleinkindes Jens G. mit der seines normal hörenden Zwillingsbruders unter besonderer Berücksichtigung ihrer sprachlichen Gestaltungskraft", Wissenschaftliche Hausarbeit Universität Hamburg Fachbereich Erziehungswissenschaft, 1961.
Gorman, P. and Paget, G. "A systematic sign language", London 1969[4].
Goto, H. "Auditory perception by normal Japanese adults of the sounds L and R", Neuropsychologica (Eng.) 1971, p. 317-323.
Granit, R. "The basis of motor control. Integrating the activity of muscles, alpha and gamma motoneurons and their leading control systems", Academic Press, London 1970.
Graser, J. B. "Der durch Gesicht- und Tonsprache der Menschheit wiedergegebene Taubstumme", Bayreuth 1829.

Graser, J. B. "Die Erziehung der Taubstummen in der Kindheit", Nürnberg 1843.

Greenstein, J. M. "Methods of Fostering Language in Deaf Infants", Final Report to Health, Education and Welfare Department, Grant OEG-0-72-539, Washington D.C. 1975.

Griffiths, C. "The utilisation of individual hearing-aids on young deaf children", Un. Southern California 1955.

Griffiths, C. "Conquering childhood deafness", New York 1967.

Groht, M. A. "Natural language for deaf children", Washington D.C. 1958.

Gross, K. and Rothenberg, S. "An examination of methods used to test the perceptual deficit hypothesis of dyslexia", Journal of Learning Disabilities 1979 (12), p. 670-677.

Guberina, P. "Verbotonal method and its application to the rehabilitation of the deaf", Proceedings Int. Congr. of Ed. of the Deaf, Washington D.C. 1963.

Guittart, P. "De intonatie van het Nederlands", Utrecht 1925.

Gutzmann, H. "Über die Sprache der Taubstummen", Medische Kliniek 1905, p. 1065-1091.

H

Hardesty, F. P. und Priester, H. J. "Hamburg-Wechsler Intelligenz Test für Kinder", Bern 1966[3].

Harris, G. M. "Language for the preschool deaf child", New York 1971[3].

Hartong, C. "Danskunst", Rotterdam 1948.

Haycock, G. S. "The teaching of speech", Stoke on Trent 1933; Washington D.C. 1954.

Hayes, C. "The ape in our house", New York 1951.

Hayes, P. M. "Feasibility of assigning deaf students to regular classes", in "Proceedings I of International Conference on oral education of the Deaf", Washington D.C. 1967, p. 406-423.

Heider, F. "A study of phonetic symbolism of deaf children", Psychological Monographs 1940 (52), p. 23-41.

Heider, F. and Heider, G. M. "Phonetic symbolism of deaf children", Volta Review 1941 (43), p. 165-168, 233-236.

Heider, F. and Heider, G. M. "Limitations of the content of communication", Psychol. Monographs 1941 (53), p. 17-29.

Helmont, F. M. van "Een zeer korte afbeelding van het ware natuurlijke Hebrewse A.B.C.", Amsterdam 1697.

Hermus, A. "Handleiding voor den aspirant doofstommenonderwijzer", St.-Michielsgestel 1927.

Higgins, P. C. "Outsiders in a hearing world. A sociology of deafness", Sage Publications, Beverly Hills, 2nd London 1980.

Hintzman, D. L. "Classification and aural coding in short term memory", Psychonomic Science 1965, p. 161-162.

Hintzman, D. L. "Articulatory coding in short-term memory", Journal of Verbal Learning and Verbal Behaviour 1967 (6), p. 312-316.

Hirsch, A. P. "Die Gebärdensprache der Hörenden und ihre Stellung zur Lautsprache. Im Anhang eine Sammlung von Hörendengebärden", Selbstverlag des Verfassers, Charlottenburg, 1923.

Hirsch, A. P. "Beobachtungen und Betrachtungen zur sprachlichen Entwicklung eines taubgeborenen Kindes", Halle (Saale) 1954.

186

Hirsh, I. J. Bilgers, R. C. and Deatherage, B. H. "The effect of auditory and visual background on apparent duration", American Journal of Psychology 1956 (69), p. 561-574.
Hiskey, M. S. "Hiskey Nebraska Test of learning aptitude", Lincoln, Nebraska 1966.
Hofmarksrichter, K. "Visuelle Kompensation und Eidetik bei Taubstummen", Archiv für die Gesammte Psychologie, Leipzig 1931.
Hofsteater, H. T. "An experiment in preschool education. An autobiographic study", 1932, Gallaudet College, Washington D.C., Bulletin no. 1, Vol. 8, 1959.
Holst, E. von und Mittelstaedt, H. "Das Reafferenz-prinzip", Naturwissenschaften 1950 (37), p. 464-476.
Holst, E. von "Relations between the central nervous system and the peripheral organs", Brit. J. Animal Behaviour 1954 (2), p. 89-94.
Houchins, R. R. "A study of some of the factors that may influence the spontaneous vocalisations of four-year-old deaf children", Dept. of Education, University of Kansas, 1954.
Hudgins, C. V. "Voice production and breath control in the speech of the deaf", Am. Annals of the Deaf 1937 (82), p. 338-363.
Hudgins, C. V. "A rationale for acoustic training", The Volta Review 1948 (59), p. 484-490.
Hudgins, C. V. "Problems of speech comprehension in deaf children", The Nervous Child 1951 (9), p. 57-63.
Hudgins, C. V. "The response of profoundly deaf children to auditory training", Journal of Speech and Hearing Disorders 1953 (18), p. 273-288.
Hudgins, C. V. "Auditory training: its possibilities and limitations", Volta Bureau, Washington D.C. 1954.
Hudgins, C. V. "Studies in the frequency discrimination of deaf children", 88 Annual Report, Clarke School for the Deaf, Northampton Mass. 1955, p. 53-55.
Hudgins, C. V. "A comparison of deaf and normal hearing subjects in the production of motor rhythms", Proceedings 38 meeting of the Conv. of Am. Inst. of the Deaf, Washington D.C. 1958, p. 200-203.
Hudgins, C. V. "The development of communication skills among profoundly deaf children in an auditory training program", in Ewing (ed.) 1960, p. 33/2-7.
Hudgins, C. V. and Numbers, F. C. "An investigation of the intelligibility of the speech of the deaf", Genet. Psych. Monographs nr. 25, 1942, p. 289-392.

I

Irwin, O. C. "Infant speech: I. Consonantal sounds according to place of articulation", Journal of Speech and Hearing Disorders 1947, p. 397-401. II. "Consonantal sounds according to manner of articulation", J.S.H.D. 1947, p. 402-404. III. "Development of vowel sounds", J.S.H.D. 1948, p. 31-34.
Irwin, R. "Speech therapy and children's linguistic skills", J.S.H.D. 1962, p. 377-381.

J

Jacobs, F. "Beiträge zum Problem des Schreiens und Lallens als unsprachliche stimmliche Äusserungen bei hörenden und hörgeschädigten Kleinkindern", Wissensch. Hausarbeit Universität Heidelberg 1968.
Jakobson, R. and Halle, M. "Fundamentals of language", Den Haag 1956.
Jeffers, J. and Barley, M. "Speechreading (lipreading)", Springfield Ill. 1971.

Johannson, H. Personal correspondence 1973.
John Tracy Clinic "Correspondence Course", Los Angelos 1973.
John, J. E. J. and Howarth, J. N. "The effect of time distortions on the intelligibility of deaf children's speech", Language and Speech 1965, p. 127-134.
Johnson, G. F. "The effects of cutaneous stimulation by speech on lipreading performance", Michigan State University 1963.
Joiner, E. "Graded lessons in speech. A manual for teachers of the deaf", Morganton N. Carolina 1936, reprint 1953.
Jussen, H. "Schwerhörige und ihre Rehabilitation" in "Sonderpädagogik 2", Ernst Klett Verlag, Stuttgart 1974, p. 185-318.

Kahn, D. and Birch, H. G. "Development of auditory-visual integration and reading achievement", Perceptual and Motor Skills 1968 (27), p. 459-468.
Kampik, A. "Experimentelle Untersuchungen über die praktische Leistungsfähigkeit der Vibrationsempfindungen", Archiv gesammte Psychologie, 1930 (76), p. 56-67.
Kampik, A. "Das Lallen beim taubgeborenen Kinde", Blätter für Taubstummenbildung 1930 (43), p. 354-356.
Kaplan, E. "Gestural representation of implement usage: an organismic developmental study", Doctoral dissertation, Clark University 1968.
Kaplan, E. "Test for apraxia", in Brown J. W. 1972, p. 157-160.
Kater, C. "Die vorsprachlichen stimmlichen Äusserungen des hörgeschädigten Kleinkindes. Eine Darstellung der Forschungen, Beobachtungen und Ansichten in der Literatur", Wissensch. Hausarbeit Universität Heidelberg, 1969.
Kates, S. L. "Learning and use of logical symbols by deaf and hearing subjects", J. abnorm. Psychol. 1969 (74), p. 699-705.
Kates, S. L. Kates, W. and Michael, J. "Cognitive processes in deaf and hearing", Psych. Monographs 1962 nr. 551.
Kates, S. L. Yudin, L. and Tiffany, R. K. "Concept attainment by deaf and hearing adolescents", J. Educ. Psych. 1962 (53), p. 119-126.
Katz, D. und Révész, G. "Musikgenuss bei Gehörlosen", Ztschr. für angewandte Psychol. 1926 nr. 99.
Keidel, W. D. "Vibrations-reception. Der Erschütterungssinn des Menschen", Erlangen 1956.
Kern, E. "Die Anbahnung der Sprachentwicklung beim taubstummen Kinde", IVe Vers. der Deutschen Gesellsch. für Sprach- und Stimmheilk., Leipzig 1934.
Kern, E. "Theorie und Praxis eines ganzheitlichen Sprach-unterrichtes für das gehörgeschädigte Kind", Freiburg 1958.
Klemm, O. "Über die Wirksamkeit kleinster Zeitunterschiede", Arch. des ges. Psychologie 1925 (50), p. 204-220.
Klima, E. S. and Bellugi, M. "Syntactic regularities in the speech of children" in Ferguson and Slobin (eds.) 1973, p. 333-354.
Klinghammer, D. "Problem der geistigen Entwicklung bei Mehrfachbehinderten", in Bodenseeländer-Tagung "Das mehrfach behinderte hörgeschädigte Kind", Bern 1971, p. 7-44.
Kloster-Jensen, M. "Un pendant à la phonématique", Universitetet i Bergen Historiskantikvarisk rekke, Norwegen 1952.
Kloster-Jensen, M. und Jussen, H. "Lautbildung bei Hörgeschädigten", Marhold, Berlin 1970.

Köble, J. "Die ersten zweieinhalb Lebensjahre eines hörgeschädigten Knaben", Wissensch. Hausarbeit Universität Heidelberg 1962.

Kohler, I. "Die Zusammenarbeit der Sinne", in "Handbuch der Psychologie", I. Band, 1. Halbband Göttingen 1966, p. 616-655.

Kolb, B. and Whishaw, I. Q. "Fundamentals of human neuropsychology", Freeman W. H. and Co, San Francisco 1980.

Kooi, D. "Leren liplezen", Amsterdam 1924.

Koppitz, E. M. "The Visual Aural Digit Span Test: experimental edition", Mount Kisco, N.Y., Koppitz 1972.

Kramar, E. J. J. and Lewis, Th. R. "Comparison of visual and non-visual listening", J. of Communication, Philadelphia 1951, p. 16-19.

Krijnen, A. "Developing the voices of very young deaf children", Proceedings of Internat. Cong. on Oral Educ. of the Deaf, Washington D.C. 1967, p. 664-671.

Krijnen, A. "Speech and speech correction for deaf children", St.-Michielsgestel 1972.

Kröhnert, O. "Die sprachliche Bildung der Gehörlosen", Verlag Julius Beltz, Weinheim 1966.

Kumpf, A. "Akustische Rückkopplung des Atemgeräusches analog dem Leeeffekt", HNO, Wegweiser für die Fachärztliche Praxis, Berlin 1964, p. 195-196.

Kwaaitaal, T. and Roskam, E. Katholieke Universiteit Nijmegen, Psychologisch Laboratorium, Personal communication 1968.

L
Lach, R. Ling, D. Ling, A. and Ship, N. "Early speech development in deaf infants", Am. Ann. 1970, p. 522-526.

Lado, R. "Language teaching. A scientific approach", New York 1964.

Lancioni, G. "Increasing the use of higher-level forms of communication in deaf children within a residential setting", The Teacher of the Deaf, 1981 (15-3), p. 77-82.

Larr, A. L. "Speechreading through closed circuit television", Volta Review 1959, p. 19-21.

Lashley, K. S. "The problem of serial order in behavior", in Jeffres L.A., New York 1951.

Lee, B. S. "Artificial stutterer", Journal of Speech and Hearing Disorders 1951, p. 53-55.

Lenneberg, E. H. "Prerequisites for language acquisition", in Proceedings of Intern. Conf. on Oral Education of the Deaf, Washington D.C. 1967, p. 1302-1361.

Lenneberg, E. H., Rebelsky, F. and Nichols, J. "The vocalisations on infants born to deaf and hearing parents", Human Development VIII no. 1, 1965, p. 23-37.

Lersch, Ph. "Aufbau der Person", J. A. Barth, München 1954, 1966[10].

Levelt, W. J. M. "The perception of syntactic structure", HB-69-30 EX, Dept. of Psychol. University Groningen 1969.

Levelt, W. J. M. "A scaling approach to the study of syntactic relations", in Flores d'Arcais and Levelt, 1970, p. 109-121.

LeZak, R. J. and Starbuck, H. B. "Identification of children with speech disorders in a residential school for the blind", The Education of the Blind U.S.A. 1964, p. 8-22.

Lieth, L. Personal correspondence 1974.

Lindner, R. "Der erste Sprachunterricht Taubstummer auf Grund statistischer, experimenteller und psychologischer Untersuchungen", Leipzig 1910.

Lindner, R. "Wiederholung eines Zeichenversuches Kerschensteiners in der Taubstummenschule", Ztschr. Paed. Psych. 1912 (13), p. 419-421.

189

Lindner, R. "Untersuchungen über die Lautsprache und ihre Anwendung auf die Pädagogik", Leipzig 1916.
Lindsay, P. H. and Norman, D. A. "Human information processing. An introduction into psychology", Academic Press, New York 1973.
Ling, D. "Three experiments on frequency transposition", Am. Annals of the Deaf 1968, p. 283-294.
Ling, D. and Doehring, D. G. "Learning limits of deaf children for coded speech", Journal of Speech and Hearing Research 1969 (12), p. 83-94.
Ling, D. and Maretic, H. "Frequency transposition in the teaching of speech to deaf children", Journal of Speech and Hearing Research 1969 (12), p. 185-192.
Ling, D. "Speech and the hearing impaired child: theory and practice", Alexander Graham Bell Association, Washington D.C. 1976.
Locke, J. L. "Short term auditory memory, oral perception and experimental sound learning", Journal of Speech and Hearing Research 1969 (12), p. 185-192.
Logger, Br. Berthilo "Ademtherapie bij pathologische gevallen", Ts. voor B.L.O. 1950, p. 104-105, 111-121, 123-130.
Lotzmann, G. (ed.) "Psychologie der Stimm-, Sprech- und Sprachrehabilitation", G. Fischer Verlag, Stuttgart 1979.
Löwe, A. "Hausspracherziehung für hörgeschädigte Kleinkinder", Berlin 1964.
Löwe, A. "Früherfassung, Früherkennung, Frühbetreuung hörgeschädigten Kinder", Berlin 1970, 2nd 1976.
Löwe, A. "Gehörlose, ihre Bildung und Rehabilitation", in "Sonderpädagogik 2", Ernst Klett Verlag, Stuttgart 1974, p. 15-171.
Lowenfeld, B. "Our blind children, growing and learning with them", Springfield Ill. 1956.
Luchsinger, R. und Arnold, G. E. "Lehrbuch der Sprach- und Stimmheilkunde", Wien 1970[4].
Luria, A. R. "Human brain and psychological processes", Harper and Row, New York 1966.
Luria, A. R. "Higher cortical functions in man", Basic Books, New York 1966.
Lutermann, D. M. "A parent centered nursery program for preschool deaf children", Office of Education (D.H.E.W.) Washington D.C., Bureau of Research, BR-6-2069, Feb. 1970, Grant OEG-1-6-062069-1591, 1970.

M
Maesse, H. "Das Verhältnis von Laut- und Gebärdensprache in der Entwicklung des taubstummen Kindes", Langensalza 1935.
Magner, M. a.o. "Speech development", Clarke School Northampton 1971.
Malisch, K. "Die Sprechempfindungen und der Sprech-unterricht bei Taubstummen", Blätter für Taubstummenbildung 1919, p. 9-24, 74-98.
Markides, A. "Home atmosphere and linguistic progress of preschool hearing handicapped children", The Teacher of the Deaf, 70, 1972, p. 7-14, 79.
Markides, A. "Comparative linguistic proficiencies of deaf children, taught by two different methods of instruction – manual versus oral", The Teacher of the Deaf, 1976, p. 307-347.
Mavilya, M. P. "Spontaneous vocalisation and babbling in hearing impaired infants", Columbia University, New York 1969.
Mavilya, M. P. "Spontaneous vocalisation and babbling in hearing impaired infants" in Fant G. (ed.) "Intern. Symposium Stockholm 1970", Washington D.C. 1972, p. 163-171.

McCarthy, D. "Language development in children" in Carmichael L. "Child psychology", London 1954², p. 492-631.

McCarty, E. L. "The relationship of various play activities to the spontaneous speech sounds of five-year old deaf children", Dept. of Education, University of Kansas U.S.A. 1954.

McGinnis, M. A. "Aphasic children, identification and education by the associative method", St. Louis 1963.

Meadow, K. P. "Early manual communication in relation to the deaf child's intellectual, social and communicative functioning", Berkeley University 1967.

Menyuk, P. "Sentences children use", M.I.T. Press, Cambridge U.S.A. 1969.

Menyuk, P. "The development of speech", Indianapolis, New York 1972.

Merken, L. "Onderzoek op geheugen van dove kinderen", Report Psychological Department of the "Instituut voor Doven" Sint-Michielsgestel, 1978.

Meumann, E. "Die Entstehung der ersten Wortbedeutungen beim Kinde", Leipzig 1902.

Millar, S. "Psychologie van het spelen", Utrecht 1970.

Miller, G. A. "The magical number seven, plus or minus two: some limits on our capacity for processing information", Psychological Review, 1956 (63), p. 81-97.

Miller, G. A. "Speech and language", in Stevens S.S. (ed.) 1960, p. 789-810.

Miller, J. "Parent education at the University of Kansas Medical Center", in "Report of Proceedings", Washington D.C. 1970, p. 318-323.

Mindel, E. D. and Vernon McCay, "They grow in silence. The deaf child and his family", Nat. Ass. of the Deaf, Silver Spring, Maryland 1971.

Mitrinovitch, A. "Modification de la respiration chez les sourds-muets atteints de troubles de la parole", Rev. Française Phoni. 1937 (5), p. 209-239.

Montpellier, G. de "Les altérations morphologiques des mouvements rapides", Louvain, Institut Supérieur de Philosophie 1933, 1935.

Moore, D. G. "Motor control in speech production", Teacher of the Deaf 1981 (5), p. 144-150.

Morsh, J. E. "A comparative study of deaf and hearing students", Am. Ann. of the Deaf 1937, p. 223-233.

Mowrer, O. H. "Learning theory and personality dynamics", New York 1950.

Mowrer, O. H. "Learning theory and symbolic process", New York 1960.

Muchow, M. Unpubl. studies on child behavior 1926 - 1930, cit. Werner H. and Kaplan B. 1963.

Mulholland, A. (ed.) "International symposium on deafness: Oral education today and tomorrow, 1979", Alexander Graham Bell Association, Washington D.C. 1980.

Müller, A. und Hägi, H. "Das Sprache-Tast-fühlen", International Congress on the care of the deaf-mute, Groningen 1950, p. 70-79.

Murray, D. J. "The role of speech responses in short term memory", Canad. Journal of Psychology 1967 (21), p. 263-276.

Murphy, L. J. and Murphy, K. P. "Tests of abilities and attainments" in Ewing A. W. G. (ed.), Manchester 1957, p. 213-234.

Myklebust, H. R. "Babbling and echolalia in language theory", Journal of Speech and Hearing Disorders 1957, p. 356-360.

Myklebust, H. R. "The psychology of deafness", New York 1964².

N

Nanninga-Boon, A. "Psychologische ontwikkelingsmethoden van het doofstomme kind", Groningen 1929.

Neas, B. J. "A study of the spontaneous babblings of three- and four-year-old deaf children" Dept. of Education, University of Kansas U.S.A. 1953.

Neppert, J. "Die Entwicklung des gehörlosen Kleinkindes Tanja D. bis zum Alter von 2;8 Jahren im Vergleich zu ihrem hörenden Zwillingsbruder, und die Darstellung der sonderpädagogischen Massnahmen. I. Teil: Von der Geburt bis zum Alter 1;11, II. Teil: Von Alter 1;11 bis 2;8", Wissenschaftliche Hausarbeit, Universität Hamburg 1969.

Neuberger, F. "Über das Lippen-lesen", Monatschrift Ohrenheilkunde 1971, p. 249-274.

Neuhaus, M. "Parental attitudes and the emotional adjustment of deaf children" Exceptional Children 1969 (35), p. 721-727.

Newman, S. S. "Further experiments in phonetic symbolism", American Journal of Psych. 1933 (45), p. 53-75.

Nober, E. H. "Cutile air and bone conduction thresholds of the deaf", Exceptional Children 1970 (36), p. 571-579.

Nober, E. H. "The development of audiologic criteria to differentiate between auditory thresholds and cutile thresholds of deaf children", Dept. of Health, Education and Welfare, U.S. Office of Education for the handicapped, Washington D.C. 1970.

Northcott, W. H. (ed.) "Curriculum guide hearing impaired children, birth to three years and their parents", UNISTAPS, Minneapolis Public School 1972.

Numbers, M. E. "The place of elements teaching in speech development", Volta Review 1942, p. 261-265.

O

Odom, P. B. Blanton R. L. and Nunnally, J. C. "Some 'cloze' technique studies of language capability in the deaf", Journal of Speech and Hearing Research 1967, p. 816-827.

Oléron, P. "Études sur le langage mimique des sourds-muets", Année Psychologique 1952 (52), p. 47-81.

Oléron, P. "Études sur le langage mimique des sourds-muets. I. Les Procédés d'expression", Année Psychologique 1953 (62), p. 47-81.

Oléron, P. "Appréhension de différences perceptives et présentation simultanée ou successive par des enfants sourds", in Revue "Defectologie" 1972 (45), p. 18-23.

Oléron, P. "Langage et développement mental", Bruxelles 1973.

Oliver, R. M. "The families of young deaf children. Experience of research in an unfamiliar field", British Journal of Psychiatric Social Work 1965 (11), p. 27-36.

O'Neill, J. J. and Oyer, H. J. "Visual communication for the hard of hearing", Englewood Cliffs, 1961 (2nd 1981).

O'Rourke, T. J. (ed.), "Psycholinguistics and total communication", Am. Ann. Washington D.C. 1972.

Overbeek, J. C. van, "Elektrische Verstärker für Taubstumme", International Congress on the Care of the Deaf-mute, Groningen 1950, p. 77-87.

Oyer, H. J. "Auditory communication for the hard of hearing", Prentice Hall Inc., Englewood Cliffs, New Jersey 1966.

Oyer, H. J. and Frankmann, J. "The aural rehabilitation process – A conceptual framework analysis", Holt, Rinehart and Winston, New York 1975.

P

Paget, R. "Education of the totally deaf", Advancement of Science 1953 (9), p. 437-441.
Parker, W. R. "Pathology of speech", New York 1951.
Paziner, K. "Der Zwillingsbruder ist taubgeboren", Hörgeschädigte Kinder 1966, p. 116-119.
Penfield, W. "The mystery of mind", Princeton 1975.
Peterson, L. R. and Johnson, S. T. "Some effects of minimising articulation on short-term retention", Journal of Verbal Language and Verbal Behaviour 1971 (10), p. 346-354.
Piaget, J. "Le langage et la pensée chez l'enfant",Neuchatel 1923.
Pickett, J. M., "Tactual communication of speech sounds to the deaf, comparison with lipreading", Journal of Speech and Hearing Disorders 1963 (28), p. 315-330.
Pickett, J. M. "Speech analysing aids", Gallaudet College, Washington D.C. 1971, p. 58-70.
Pickett, J. M. and Pickett, B. H. "Communication of speech sounds by a tactual vocoder", Journal of Speech and Hearing Research 1963, p. 207-222.
Pickless, A. M. "Hometraining with hearing-aids" in Ewing (ed.) 1957, p. 77-104.
Postma, C. G. "Voorschool en articulatie-onderwijs", Ned. Tijdschr. voor Doofstommenonderwijs 1936.
Povel, D. J. "Evaluation of the vowel corrector in the practice of the speech training of deaf boys", Kath. Univers. Nijmegen, Psychologisch Laboratorium 1974.
Prick, J. J. G. "De invloed van afwijkende motoriek op het geheel der persoonlijkheid, mede in verband met de indicatie tot bewegingstherapie", Ned. Tijdschr. v. Geneeskunde 1959, p. 489-495.
Prick, J. J. G. en Calon, P. J. A. "Het aphasie-probleem na 125 jaar", Ned. Tijdschr. Psych. 1950, p. 369-400.
Prick, J. J. G. and Calon, P. J. A. "Een schets van intelligentie en dementie", Amsterdam 1967.
Prick, J. J. G. and Van der Waals, H. G. "Nederlands handboek der psychiatrie", deel I en III, Arnhem 1958, 1965.

Q

Quigley, S. P. "The influence of fingerspelling on the development of language, communication and educational achievement in deaf children", Urbana, Univ. of Illinois 1969.

R

Rapin, J., Costa, L. D., Mandel, I. J. and Fromowitz, A. J. "Keytapping and delayed feedback", Journal of Speech and Hearing Research 1966, p. 278-288.
Rau, E. F. "Methods of educating very young deaf children", Volta Review 1935 (37), p. 514-518, 579-583, 649-654, 700-701.
Redgate, G. W. Palmer, J. Wilkins, C. G. Smart, C. A. M. and Black, E. "The teaching of reading to deaf children. An experimental study", Manchester University, Dept. of aud. and Ed. of the Deaf, 1972.
Reichling, A. "A new method of speech training in deaf-mutism", Proceedings II Intern. Congress for maladjusted children, Amsterdam 1949.
Reichling, A. "Het woord", Utrecht 1935, herdruk 1967.
Reichling, A. "Verzamelde studies over hedendaagse problemen der taalwetenschap", Zwolle 1969[5].

Remlein-Mozalewska, G. "Das Sehen im Leben des hörgeschädigten Kindes", Hörgeschädigte Kinder 1980 (17), p. 146-152.
Révèsz, G. "Die Formenwelt des Tastsinnes", Martinus Nijhoff, Den Haag 1938.
Révèsz, G. "Inleiding tot de muziekpsychologie", Amsterdam 1946.
Rieder, O. "Die vorsprachlichen stimmlichen Äusserungen", Universität Heidelberg 1963.
Rileigh, K. K. and Odom, P. B. "Perception of rhythm by subjects with normal and deficient hearing", Dev. Psychol. 1972, p. 54-61.
Ringel, R. L. House, A. S. Buck, K. W. Dolinski, J. P. and Scott, C. M. "Some relations between orosensory discrimination and articulatory aspects of speech production", Journal of Speech and Hearing Disorders 1970 (35), p. 3-11.
Ringel, R. L. and Steer, M. D. "Some effects of tactile and auditory alterations on speech output", Journal of Speech and Hearing Research 1963, p. 369-378.
Riper, C. van "Speech correction: principles and methods", Englewood Cliffs N. J. 1954.
Risberg, A. "Recording of speech for the deaf", preliminary report Royal Institute of Technology, Stockholm 1964.
Rogers, M. 1867, in Yale C. A., "Formation and development of elementary English sounds", Northampton Mass. Clarke School for the Deaf 1938.
Rosenstein, J. "Tactile perception of rhythmic patterns by normal, blind, deaf and aphasic children", Am. Annals of the Deaf 1957 (102), p. 399-403.
Rosenstein J., "Cognitive abilities of deaf children", Journal of Speech and Hearing Research 1960, p. 108-119.
Rosenstein, J. "Perception, cognition and language in deaf children", Exceptional Children 1960-1961, p. 276-284.
Ross, A. O. "Psychological aspects of learning disabilities and reading disorders", McGraw Hill, New York 1976.
Ruesch, J. and Kees, W. "Nonverbal communication", Berkeley 1956.
Rutten F. J. Th., Personal communication, Annual Report St. Michielsgestel 1941.
Rutten, F. J. Th. e.a., "Menselijke verhoudingen", Bussum ·1956².
Rutten F. J. Th., "Stervende taal", Film and Manual, Stichting Film en Wetenschap, Utrecht 1957.

S
Sanden, A. L. M. van der, "Het analyseren van strukturele verandering. Een methodologische aantekening ten behoeve van de ontwikkelingspsychologie", Kath. Universiteit Nijmegen, Groep Ontwikkelingspsychologie 1973.
Sanden, A. L. M. van der, Personal communication 1974.
Sanden, P. van de, "Verslag van didactische hulp aan een 19-jarige dove jongen met gebrekkige vooropleiding", Kath. Leergangen, Tilburg 1974.
Sands, E. S. Freeman, F. J. and Harris, K. S. "Progressive changes in articulatory patterns in verbal apraxia: a longitudinal case study", Brain and Language 1978 (6), p. 97-105.
Sapir, E. "A study of phonetic symbolism", J. exper. Psychology 1929 (12), p. 225-239.
Satz, P. and Nostrand, G. K. van, "Developmental dyslexia: an evaluation of a theory", in Satz and Ross (eds.) 1973, p. 121-148.
Satz, P. and Ross, J. (eds), "The disabled learner: early detection and intervention", Universitaire Pers Rotterdam, Swets and Zeitlinger, Lisse 1973.
Schär, A. "Untersuchungen über die Tonhöhe-bewegungen in der Sprache der

Taubstummen", Vox 1921, p. 62-80.
Schiff, W. and Dytell, R. S. "Deaf and hearing children's performance on a tactual perception battery", Perceptual and Motor Skills 1972 (36), p. 683-706.
Schlesinger, H. S. and Meadow, K. P. "Sound and sign. Childhood deafness and mental health", Un. of California Press, Berkeley 1972.
Schorsch, E. (ed), "Handbuch des Taubstummenwesens", Osterwieck am Harz, 1929.
Schulte, K. "Vibrative Sprechgliederungshilfe für Sprach-taube", Neue Bl. Taubstummenbildung 1969, p. 72-77.
Schulte, K. "Das Fonator-System und sein Einsatz als Sprechgliederungshilfe bei gehörlosen Kindern", Hörgeschädigte Kinder 1972 (9), p. 60-64.
Schulte, K. und Roessler, H. "Optische Phonemdarstellung als Sprechgliederungshilfe für hörgeschädigte Kinder", Neckar Verlag, Villingen 1971.
Schumann, P. "Geschichte des Taubstummenwesens", Frankfurt a.M. 1940.
Schuy, Cl. "Die sprachliche Situation der Taubstummen", Sprachforum 1955, p. 146-160.
Scott, C. M. and Ringel, R. L. "Articulation without oral sensory control", Journal of Speech and Hearing Research 1971, p. 804-818.
Seashore, C. E. "Psychology of music", New York 1938.
Senf, G. M. "An information-integration theory and its application to normal reading acquisition and reading disability", in Bryant and Kass (eds.).
Simmons, A. A. "Language growth through lipreading" in "Proceedings of the Intern. Congress of Ed. of the Deaf", Washington D.C. 1964, p. 333-338.
Simmons-Martin, A. "The oral/aural procedure. Theoretical basis and rationale", Volta Review 1972, p. 541-551.
Skinner, B. F. "Verbal behavior", London 1957.
Sleigh, P. "A study of some symbolic processes in young children", Brit. J. Disorders of Communication 1972 (7), p. 163-175.
Smith, F. "Understanding reading. A psycholinguistic analysis of reading and learning to read", Ndw York 1971.
Smith, O. W. and Koutstaal, C. W. "Some correlates of language distance and their factor structure", Percept. and Motor Skills 1970, p. 207-210.
Smits, L. F. M. "Video en liplezen; beschrijving en evaluatie van een experimentele oefenmethode tot verbetering van de gespreksvaardigheid van oudere dove kinderen", Sint-Michielsgestel 1975.
Snijders, J. Th. and Snijders-Oomen, A. W. M. "Niet-verbaal intelligentieonderzoek van horenden en doofstommen", Groningen 1958, 2nd 1961, 1970.
Speth, Br. Leo, "Adem en accent", St.-Michielsgestel 1958.
Stambak, M. "Épreuves de niveau et de style moteurs" in Zazzo R. (ed.) "Manuel pour l'examen psychologique de l'enfant" nr. 2, Neuchatel 1965.
Stark, R. E. "The use of real-time visual displays of speech in the training of a profoundly deaf, nonspeaking child: a case report", Journal of Speech and Hearing Disorders 1971, p. 397-409.
Stern, C. und Stern, W. "Die Kindersprache", Leipzig 1907, 1928[4].
Stern, W. "Allgemeine Psychologie auf personalistischer Grundlage", Den Haag 1935.
Sterritt, G. M. Camp, B. W. and Lipman, B. S. "Effects of early auditory deprivation upon auditory and visual information processing", Perceptual and Motor Skills 1966, p. 123-130.
Stevens, L. M. "Curriculum Schoolrijpheid. Deel III Een evaluatieonderzoek", Malmberg, 's-Hertogenbosch 1975.

Stevens, S. S. "Handboek of experimental psychology", New York, Wiley 1960.
Stokoe W. C., "Semiotics and human sign languages", The Hague 1972.
Straus, E. "Vom Sinn der Sinne", Berlin 1956.
Stritzver, G. L. "Frequency discrimination of deaf children and its relationship to their achievement in auditory training", Volta Review 1958 (60), p. 304-306.
Stuckless, E. R. (ed.) "INFO series 3, a review of research at National Technical Institute for the Deaf 1967 – 1976", National Technical Institute for the Deaf, Rochester N.Y. 1978.
Stuckless, E. R. and Birch, J. W. "The influence of early manual communication on the linguistic development of deaf children", Am. Ann. of the Deaf 1966, p. 452-460, 499-504 (Final Report Min. of Education, Health and Welfare, Washington D.C. 1964).
Stuckless, E. R. and Subtelny, J. D. "Research on communication and deafness", Proceedings of the Conference of Executives of American Schools for the Deaf, Rochester N.Y. 1976.
Sumby, W. H. and Pollack I. , "Visual contribution to speech intelligibility in noise", Journal of the Acoustical Society of America, 1954, p. 212-215.
Sykes, J. L. "A study of the spontaneous vocalisations of young deaf children", Psychological Monograph: Studies in the psychology of the deaf, 1940 (52), p. 104-123.

T

Taaffe, G. "The cognitive structure of lipreading", Wayne State University, Department of Education and Psychology 1968.
Taaffe, J. and Wong, W. "Studies of variables in lipreading stimulus material", John Tracy Clinic Research papers III, Los Angelos 1957.
Taylor, G. "Basic problems in the mental health of preschool deaf children" in Ewing (ed.) 1960, p. 57/1-4.
Teel, J. Winston, M. Aspinall, K. Rousey, C. and Goetzinger, C. P. "Thresholds of hearing by respiration using a polygraph", Arch. Otolar. 1967, p. 172-174.
Templin, M. "Certain language skills in children", Institute of Child Welfare Monograph nr. 26, Minneapolis, Minnesota 1957.
Templin, M. C. and Darley, F. L. "The Templin Darley test of articulation", Iowa City, Univ. Iowa Bureau Educational Res. and Sci., Extension Div. 1960.
Tervoort, B. "Structurele analyse van visueel taalgebruik binnen een groep dove kinderen", Amsterdam 1953.
Tervoort, B. Geest A. J. M. v.d., Hubers G. A. C., Prins R. S. en Snow C. E., "Psycholinguistiek", Utrecht 1972.
Tervoort, B. and Verberk, A. J. A. "Final report on project number R.D.-467-64-65 of the vocational rehabilitation administration of the Department of Health, Education and Welfare, Washington D.C. titled: Analysis of communicative structure patterns", 1967, Den Haag 1974.
Thomassen, A. J. W. M. "On the representation of verbal items in short term memory", Kath. Universiteit, Psych. Lab., Nijmegen 1970.
Thompson, R. F. "Introduction to physiological psychology", Harper and Row, New York 1975.
Tinker, M. A. Hackner, F. and Wesley, M. W. "Speed and quality of assocation as a measure of vocabulary knowledge", J. Educ. Psychol. 1940 (31), p. 575-582.
Travis, L. E. (ed.), "Handbook of speech pathology and audiology", New York 1971.

U

Uden, A. van, "Voelmuziek en dans voor doofstommen", St.-Michielsgestel 1947.
Uden A. van, "Een geluidsmethode voor zwaar- en geheel dove kinderen", St.-Michielsgestel 1952.
Uden, A. van, "Inleidende proef met blaasorgeltjes", Tijdschrift voor Doofstommenonderwijs 1955, p. 32-37.
Uden, A. van, "Taalonderwijs en hoortraining", St.-Michielsgestel 1955.
Uden, A. van en Uden, L. van, "Het behoeden voor verstomming. Hometraining", St.-Michielsgestel 1957.
Uden, A. M. J. van, "Erfahrungsbericht über drei Jahre Hauserziehung tauber Kleinkinder", Neue Blätter für Taubstummenbildung, 1959 (13), p. 76-82.
Uden, A. van, "A sound perceptive method" in Ewing (ed.) 1960, p. 19/3-12.
Uden, A. van, "Gehörlosenschule und Schwerhörigenschule als verschiedene Schultypen", N.Bl.T.Bi. 1960, p. 161-173.
Uden, A. van, "Spraak-verstaan", Methode om technische verstaansvaardigheid van dove kinderen te meten, St.-Michielsgestel 1962, p. 45-53.
Uden, A. M. J. van, "Instructing prelingually deaf children by rhythm of bodily movements and of sounds, by oral mime and general bodily expression, – its possibilities and difficulties", in: Proc. int. congr. educ. of the deaf, Washington 1963.
Uden, A. M. J. van, "Der Rhythmus bei der Hörerziehung gehörloser Kinder. Theorie und Praxis, besonders bei der Hausspracherziehung und im Kindergarten", in: Arbeitstagung für Hörerziehung 1968-1969, Erlangen 1971.
Uden, A. M. J. van, "Eupraxie en spraak", Sint-Michielsgestel 1970.
Uden, A. van, "Het ritme bij de hoortraining van prelinguaal gehoorgestoorde kinderen. Theorie en praktijk, speciaal bij de hometraining en in de voorschool. Een programma voor ritmiek bij de hometraining en in de voorschool", Het Gehoorgestoorde Kind 1971, p. 129-143.
Uden, A. van "Taalverwerving door taalarme kinderen", Rotterdam 1973.
Uden, A. van, "Over dove kleuters. Zeven studies met notities en literatuur-opgave", St.-Michielsgestel 1973.
Uden, A. M. J van, "Dove kinderen leren spreken", University-Press, Rotterdam, 1974.
Uden, A. M. J. van, "A world of language for deaf children. Part I: Basic Principles. A maternal reflective method", Rotterdam 1968, 3rd Lisse 1977.
Uden, A. M. J. van, "How to come into conversation with a still speechless and languageless child", Sint-Michielsgestel, St. Louis 1978.
Uden, A. M. J. van, "Diagnose von solchen Hirnstörungen, die die rein lautsprachliche Erziehung von gehörlosen Kindern gefährden", – "Diagnosis of such learning disabilities, which endanger the purely oral education of deaf children", Proceedings Hamburg 1980, J. Groos Verlag, Heidelberg 1982.
Uden, A. M. J. van, "Het belang van geheugentraining", Van Horen Zeggen 1980 (21), p. 52-64.
Uden, A. M. J. van, "Geheugentraining in de praktijk bij gehoorgestoorde, inclusief spraaktaal-gestoorde kinderen", Van Horen Zeggen, 1981 (22), p. 99-106.

V

Vahle, H. "Der Sprachunterricht" in Bund Deutscher Taubstummenlehrer "Handbuch des Taubstummenwesens", Osterwieck am Harz 1929, p. 198-393.
Vannes, G. "Vocabulaire de base du Néérlandais", Antwerpen 1962.

Vatter, J. "Die Ausbildung des Taubstummen in der Lautsprache" I II III, Frankfurt a.M. 1891-1899.
Veldt, J. v.d. "L'apprentissage du mouvement et l'automatisme", Leuven 1928.
Vellutino, F. R. "Alternative conceptualizations of dyslexia: Evidence in support of a verbal deficit hypothesis", Harvard Educational Review, 1977 (47), p. 334-354.
Verbist, A. "De psychologie van het toontreffen", De Moderne School 1933.
Vernon, M. and Koh, S. D. "Effects of early manual communication on achievement of deaf children", Am. Annals of the Deaf 1970, p. 527-536.
Vester, F. "Denken, Lernen, Vergessen", Deutsche Verlagsanstalt GmbH, Stuttgart 1975.
Vester, F. "Phänomen Stress", Deutscher Taschenbuch Verlag, München 1978.
Voorhoeve, P. E. Walter W. G. and Brink G. v.d., "Physiologie van het centrale zenuwstelsel en de zintuigen", Amsterdam 1971.

W

Walther, E. "Handbuch der Taubstummenbildung", Berlin 1895.
Wechsler, D. "Wechsler intelligence scale for children", The Psychological Corporation, New York 1949.
Wechsler, D. "Wechsler preschool and primary scale of intelligence", The Psychological Corporation, New York 1967.
Wedenberg, E. "Auditory training of deaf and hard-of-hearing children", Stockholm 1951.
Weiner, P. S. "Auditory discrimination and articulation", Journal of Speech and Hearing Disorders 1967, p. 19-28.
Weir, R. H. "Language in the crib", Den Haag 1962.
Wells, J. "The Paget systematic sign language. The use of a manual method for accelerating the development of oral language in young deaf children", T. of the Deaf 1972, p. 28-39.
Werd, Zr. Rosa de, "Iets uit de praktijk van het spreekonderwijs aan dove kinderen", St.-Michielsgestel 1949, 1964.
Werner, H. "Einführung in die Entwicklungspsychologie", München 1928, 1959[4].
Werner H. and Kaplan B., "Symbol formation", New York 1963.
Whitacker, H. A. and Noll, J. D. "Some linguistic parameters of the Token Test", Neuropsychologia, 1972 (10), p. 395-404.
White, A. H. "The effects of Total Communication, manual communication, oral communication and reading on the learning of factual information in residential school for the deaf", Michigan State University, Department of Special Education, Michigan 1972.
White, B. L. Castle P. and Held R., "Observations on the development of visually directed reading", in Hellmuth J. "Exceptional infant", Vol. I, New York 1964.
White, B. L. and Held, R. "Plasticity of sensorimotor development in the human infant" in Rosenblith J. and Allenswith W. "The causes of behavior: readings in child development and educational psychology", Boston 1966.
Wickelgren, W. A. "Distinctive features and errors in short-term-memory for English vowels", Journal of the Acoustical Society of America 1965 (38), p. 583-588.
Wickelgren, W. A. "Distinctive features and errors in short-term-memory for English consonants", Journal of the Acoustical Society of America 1966 (38), p. 388-398.

Wiener, M. Derve S., Rubinow S. and Geller J., "Nonverbal behavior and nonverbal communication", Psychol. Review 1972, p. 185-214.
Willemain, T. R. and Lee, F. F. "Tactile pitch feedback for deaf speakers", Volta Review 1971, p. 541-553.
Wing, H. "Tests of musical ability and appreciation. An investigation into the measurement, distribution and development of musical capacity", Cambridge 1968.
Wissen, I. and Blesalski, P. "Das Frostig-Programm in der klinischen Anwendung bei visuellen Wahrnehmungsstörungen sprachgestörter und hörgeschädigter Kinder", Folia Phoniatrica 1977 (29), p. 109-118.
Withrow, F. "Immediate memory span of deaf and normally hearing children", Exceptional Children 1968 (35), p. 33-41.
Woldring, S. "Over de ademhaling tijdens het spreken van dove kinderen", Ned. Tijdschrift voor Doofstommenonderwijs 1956, p. 153-160.
Wong, B. "The role of theory in learning disabilities research. Part II. A Selective review of current theories of learning and reading disabilities", Journal of Learning Disabilities 1979 (12), p. 649-658.
Woodward, M. E. and Barber, C. G. "Phoneme perception in lipreading", Journal of Speech and Hearing Research 1960 (3), p. 212-222.
Woodworth, R. S. and Schlosberg, H. Rev. ed. Kling J. W. and Riggs, L. A. "Experimental psychology", London 1971[4].
Wyke, M. A. (ed.) "Developmental aphasia", Academic Press, London 1978.

Y
Yale, C. A. "Formation and development of elementary English sounds", Northampton Mass. Clarke School for the Deaf 1938.
Young, E. H. and Hawk, S. S. "Moto-kinesthetic speech training", Stanford California 1938.
Youniss, J. and Furth, H. G. "The influence of transitivity on learning in hearing and deaf children", Child Development 1965 (36), p. 535-538.
Youniss, J. and Furth, H. G. "The role of language and experience on the use of logical symbols", Br. J. of Psychology 1967 (58), p. 435-443.
IJsseldijk, F. "Sociale ontwikkelingsaspecten bij jeugdige doven", Universiteit Nijmegen, Psych. Lab. 1971.

Z
Zaliouk, A. "Falsetto-voice in deaf children", Curr. Probl. Phon. Logop. 1960 (1), p. 217-219.
Zazzo, R.; Gallifret-Granjon, N.; Mathon, T. and Stambak, M. " Manuel pour l'examen psychologique de l'enfant", Paris 1964.

Alphabetic index

206

Luterman, D. M.   47

Malisch, K.   52
Markides, A.   32, 47, 49
Mason Publishing Company Paris   84
mathematical operation   37
Mavilya, M. P.   39, 40
McCarty, E. L.   41
McGinnis, M. A.   11
Meadow, K. P.   47
melody   27
memory   1, 3, 4, 7, 8, 21, 23, 26, 28,
    31, 32, 33, 35, 36, 38, 51, 72, 81,
    119, 120, 135-140, 147, 176
    – and activiness   120, 139-140
    auditory –   7, 26, 28, 32
    cognitive –, conative –, motor
    –   33
    "– for colours"-test   81, 119
    see *test*
    "echoic –"   137
    – for geometric figures   119, 147
    – for graphic words   35, 38, 119,
    138
    – for idioms   137-138
    intermodal –   33
    intramodal –   33
    motor –   21
    – for "non-pictorial words"   119
    see *test*
    – for pictures   119
    – profile   33, 72
    – as "retrieval function"   33
    – for simultaneously and succes-
    sively presented visual data   58,
    116, 117, 119, 135-136, 138, 139-
    140
    – and "set"   135-137
    short and long term –   35
    – for speech   51, 72, 137-138,
    176
    – for spoken sentences   72, 137-
    138
    see *test*
    visual –   8
    – for words   36
mental deficiency   3
"mental pictures"   174
mental training   173-174

Menyuk, P.   27, 41
Merken, L.   13, 119
methods of teaching speech   51 sqq.,
    73
    "eclectic" way of –   55
    analytic –, "Kern" –, "moulding"
    –, "prefab" –, "reactive" –, syn-
    thetic –, "Tadoma" –   52-54
    – and various degrees of transiti-
    vity   54
"Metropolitan Paragraph Reading"-
    test   134
    see *test*
Miller, G.   45
Miller, J.   41, 45
Mindel, E. D.   39
"Minimal Brain Dysfunction"
    (MBD)   34
mirror for teaching speech   26, 55,
    145, 173-174
Mitrinovitch, A.   48
Mittelstaedt, H.   145
mnesia   6
monitoring point to point –   23
Montpellier, G. de   26, 173
Moore, D. G.   29
"Moro-reflex"   27
Morsch, J. E.   48
motivation   31, 32, 139-140, 174
mother-child   27
    interaction of –   27
    speech of –   27
motor-dysphasia-aphasia   48, 72, 138
    see *euphasia*
Motor function   1, 3, 8, 12, 20, 21,
    22-23, 26, 27, 31, 33, 38, 40, 48,
    52, 54, 72, 116, 117, 123, 135-
    137, 173
    see *body-scheme, eupraxia*
    automation of –   173
    – and brain   21
    complexity of –   23
    control of –   8, 23, 33, 173-174
    coordination, sequencing, rhythm,
    planning of –   21
    expressive –   31
    fine –, gross –, fluent –   116, 117,
    123, 135
    Gestaltformation of –   21, 26, 52

210

213

brain 4, 6, 39 sqq., 137-138
– by reverse imitation 52
– as rhythmic behaviour "par ex-
cellence" 51
rhythm of – 51, 176
routine in – 49, 142
– and sensory impressions 53
see *control*
data of Sint Michielsgestel
58 sqq.
steering of – 49
see *control, steering*
"supple use of the mouth" 69,
116
syllabication of – 52
tempo of – 62, 176
– therapist 49
basic rule of training – 54
– and motor transitivity 53, 54
see *intransitivity, transitivity*
– and video-set 145-146
visual control of – 145
see *control*
visualisation of own – 146, 173-
174
see *control*
spelling of vowels 36
Spe.rep.
"Repetition of imitated words"-
test 105
see *test*
Speth, L. 48
spondee-test 137
see *test*
sport 174
Stambak, M. 124
Stanton, D. A. G. 48
Steer, M. D. 35
"steering"-functions 23, 24, 25, 26,
38, 49
anticipatory – 26
associative – 26
"considering function" of – 26
"– from point to point" 25
– of speech 49
Stern, W. 20
Sterrit, G. M. 48
Stevens, L. M. 77
"stimulogeneous fibrillation" 19

stimulus-response function 19, 28
stochastic function 19
Stuckless, E. R. 16
subcortical functions 31
see *cortical functions*
sub-Gestalts, hierarchy of – 23, 26,
31
Su.Fo.
"Paperfolding"-test 81-82
see *test*
Su.Pi.
"Visual Attention Span" in a successive way 82
"supple use of the mouth when speaking" 69, 116, 140
Sykes, J. L. 40, 41
synapsis 19
"Syndrome of dyspraxia" 9-10, 58,
70, 76, 79 sqq., 135-136, 141-142
treatment of – 10

tachypnoea 48
"tactile oral stereognosis" 35
tactual sense 20, 26, 32, 34, 35, 53
impression of speech 53
see *kineme*
"Tad-Oma"-method of speech training 53
"Tast-Fühl-Struktur" 11
Taylor, G. 46
teachers, ability and continuity of
– 47, 70, 80
"technical communicative ability" 66-
68
Teel, J. 48
telephone, graphic – 16
television 16
tempo 26, 48, 72, 139, 173-174
see *speech, motor function*
– of conversation 173-174
– of deaf children 139
terminology, tripartite – 24
test
"Bead Patterns"-test 74
"Block Patterns"-test 74
"coding"-test 82-83
"Completion of Drawings"-
test 74
correlation of eupraxia tests with

Wechsler I.Q., hearing loss and speech hearing 139-140
"Digit-Span"-test 63, 69, 82
"Digit-symbol-association"-test 139
"Eighteen syllable sentence"-test 63
"Finger-position"-test 123, 133-134
"Finger Movement"-test 91-96, 123
"Geometric figure drawing"-test 83, 147
"Geometric figure identification"-test 83
"Imitation of gestures"-test 84-91
"Intermodal integration"-test for deaf preschool children 97-99
"Intermodal integration"-test for deaf children of 6-12 years of age 103-104
"Knox' cube"-test 84, 147
"Lipreading-Hearing-Imitating"-test 63, 66-68, 104, 123-124, 134-135, 137, 175-176
"Memory for colours"-test 74, 81, 119
"Memory of geometric figures"-test 119
"Memory of non-pictorial words"-test 119
"Metropolitan Paragraph Reading"-test 134
"Nebraska-Hiskey test of Learning Aptitude" 73-74
"One Minute Reading Aloud"-test 147
"Oral fluency"-test 66-68, 104, 133-134, 138, 146
"Paper folding" 74, 81-82
"Picture Association"-test 74
"Picture Identification"-test 74
"Rhythm"-test 71, 91, 96-104, 123-124, 140
"Rhythm test for deaf preschool children" 96-100, 133
"Rhythm test for deaf children of 6-12 year of age" 100-102

"Repetition of correctly imitated words"-test 66-69, 105, 137-138, 147
"Snijders-Oomen non-verbal intelligence"-test, S.O.N.-test 146
"Speech memory"-test 73
"Spondee"-test 137
"Visual Attention Span" 74, 82, 119, 139-140
"Visual Attention Span"-test, simultaneous versus successive presentation 139-140
"Wechsler Intelligence"-test 134
testing deaf children, peculiarities of – 105
test-tape for lipreading 152 sqq.
Thomassen, A. J. W. M. 63
Thompson, R. F. 19
threshold loss of perception 34
Tinker, M. A. 134
"Token"-test 7
training 38, 146, 155, 166, 167, 173-174
    active and passive – 38
    conscious and unconscious effects of – 146
    mental – 173-174
    – and number of trials 167
    transfer of – 38, 155, 166
transitivity of speech movement 53
"triggering effect" 25, 26
tripartite terminology 24
typewriting 11, 35, 36

Uden, A. M. J. van 11, 24, 33, 41, 42, 45, 48, 51, 52, 56, 58, 63, 73, 76, 79, 86, 91, 92, 93, 96, 104, 119, 123, 124, 138

Vahle, H. 173, 174
Vatter, J. 11, 52
Vellutino, F. R. 7
Veldt, J. van der 26, 173
ventricles, enlarged – 25
verbal ability 138
    see "Oral fluency"
verbal intelligence 134
    see intelligence
verbalisation of activities 38

215